VIRTUAL REALITY: FUTURE OF HEALTH CARE

VIRTUAL REALITY: FUTURE OF HEALTH CARE

Lynne Edgar

Thesis Project

*Submitted in fulfillment
of the requirements for the degree of
Master of Business Administration*

CENTURY UNIVERSITY

iUniverse, Inc.
New York Lincoln Shanghai

VIRTUAL REALITY: FUTURE OF HEALTH CARE

iUniverse, Inc.

For information address:
iUniverse, Inc.
2021 Pine Lake Road, Suite 100
Lincoln, NE 68512
www.iuniverse.com

ISBN: 0-595-29644-0

THE FINAL PROJECT
OF
LYNNE S. EDGAR

_____

_____

_____

Contents

SPECIAL ACKNOWLEDGMENT

Michael Robbins, M.D.
Neurological Surgeon
Chair
Mercy General Hospital
Sacramento, California

ABSTRACT

OF

VIRTUAL REALITY:
FUTURE OF HEALTH CARE

by
Lynne Edgar

The problem addressed is research and development breakthroughs require a better understanding of health care medical practices. This research was to assess, review, and investigate industries of high technical research to apply intervention of improved medical treatments and diagnosis.

A sample of tomorrow's technology started several years ago in research labs exploring new technology. Research universities receive the largest federal grants grossing $483 million dollars in the fiscal year 1997 promising procurement of space technology in medicine. Through effective integration, phototype surgical room and other such visionary diffusion of technology focuses on the growth and development for the future of world medicine to global access.

Hospital groups differ on interventions for tomorrow's medicine. 3-D interface, volume reconstruction, virtual imagery, stealth platform surgery guided systems all enhance conventional medicine in treatment planning, diagnostic tests and surgical interventions. Consolidating services, acquiring contracts and partnerships in medicine, DNA therapies, molding bone for reconstruction, developing tissue replacement, and cloning organs provide good outcomes in patient care.

Recommendations include implementing a number of affordable telemedicines to attract more physician based hospital practice and use video interactive remote systems as fluoroscopy and computerized scanning to lead to the next door-surgical procedures aided via artificial intelligence. Research provided a broad mission of bio-medical research focusing on nanotechnology, artificial-aided intelligence for smart rooms, surgical-angio suites, and main centers to allow private medical sector to perform better in the highly competitive market. The National Institute of Health (NIH) supports clinical trials to determine the safety and efficiency of the new health care interventions. The National Library of Medicine (NLM) supports the evaluation used in telemedicine, MEDLARS, MEDLINE, and Health Star Interventions.

1

INTRODUCTION

STATEMENT OF THE PROBLEM

Research and development is too slow. The purpose of this study was to assess, review, and investigate high technology systems used in health care industry.

In the New Millennium, scientific research captures the dawn. Solid proof, not conjecture, will entrap reserved advances in medicine. Research is powerful enough to use new technologies to expand and to direct monies in health care institutions (Strauss, J., 1998).

Research is like three blind men feeling their way around an elephant. One blind man holding the tail, thought the elephant was long and skinny, like a snake. The second blind man, touching the elephant's side, thought the elephant was solid and big like a wall. The third blind man, holding the trunk, thought the elephant was a hose. If the three blind men could see the elephant they would know what it is and decide whether to climb the elephant's back or to step out of its way to avoid being trampled. Research has removed the blindfold. Until now, health care professionals have lived as automatons, blindly obeying decrepit mandates. Clinging to the old medical procedures, causing administrative damage on business, government and society. Choosing inventiveness in technology, signifies the exploration beyond today's limited resources, traveling into realms of knowledge to nurture, to survive and to thrive in health care.

Rather than just seeing the potential benefits, medical research has provided insight and emergence of high technological systems for medical diagnosis and treatment.

The rehearsal is over. We are a society headed to a global village. It is no surprise that computers have dominated the twentieth century in medicine. Computers have enhanced societies capacity for knowledge and connects medical institutions as units, shrinking borders bringing Marshall McLuhan's concept of a "global village" to forefront (Martinez, R., Ph.D., 1994).

1

Society is interconnected through computers. Computer networks that span the world and speeds us into the information revolution. Easing our access to knowledge, computers are used to redefine our social, political and economic structures. Every man and child uses a computer to reach across the globe for information, research and solutions for mankind.

Many administrators and health care providers, as well as patients, feel that the most pressing problem related to hospitalization are the increasing barriers that block access to health care. (Aday, 1984; Millanan, 1993; Callahan & David, 1995). Barriers to access may be grouped into broad categories: a) inability to pay, b) sociocultural obstacles to care, and organizational problems with structure of other health care delivery systems, and c) increasingly many Americans are either uninsured or underinsured, leading to delays in seeking preventive comprehensive services from a primary care provider, which then contributes to excess morbidity (Callahan & David, 1995).

Cutting costs again remains a primary objective. Researchers argue that new technology will supply advanced systems to meet cost cutting goals (Bensen, 1995). Utilization of high tech medical devices will decrease hospitalization stay and would reduce hospital costs. Reduction of staff for patient care would be lower. The surgical operation reduces cost. Benefits are not purely financial because hospitals will compete on the basis of cost, quality, customer satisfaction and positive outcomes of long-term value and depth and breathe (Aday, I., 1993).

IMPORTANCE OF THE PROBLEM

The average hospital is falling behind competitive standards (The Rising Tide, 1996, The Advisory Board Company). The Advisory Board Company has investigated the competitive standards throughout the United States. The outcome for hospitals remains to be seen. Increasing demands on continuing education strikes worldwide concern while decreasing cost remains a competitive strategy. The learning curve for new technology advances will serve as a benchmark for positive outcomes.

Acquisition of visual equipment, like biomedical libraries, will introduce physicians, nurses, technologists to the next step of medicine. The Stealth Platform is an example of medical practices that the Advisory Board Company recommends for rapid implementation of programs for future competitive edge. Surgical-angio suites of tomorrow will comply with its expectations (Surgical Navigator Technologies, 1997).

In a darkened, 40-seat theater on the UCLA campus, researchers representing a wide variety of fields are coming together immersed in virtual reality. On the giant spherical-shaped screen facility known as Visualization Portal, a physicist can display larger-than-life simulation of laser-plasma interaction. Cardiology researchers can view a fibrillating heart, a classics professor can explore the archaeological sites around the word—virtually speaking—through the use of 3-P computer models (Taubes, G., 2000).

The portal, conceived by the campus Office of Academic Computing, is currently the only university-based facility of its kind in the West. "This will be a tool to help researchers understand their own work better and explore new possibilities as well as enable them to show their work to potential donors, funding agencies and provide innovative instructions to students," explains Margo Reveil, coordinator of the Visualization Portal.

The facility is equipped with high-end work stations, hardware and software from Apple, SGI, CISCO and IBM. An immersive, virtual-reality display provided by Trimenson Systems, providing overlapping and blended images that can be displayed as a single image across the 8-foot by 24-foot curved screen. The portal is connected remotely to a network of labs throughout UCLA. "The idea is to serve as an entryway to UCLA research and instruction," says Paul Hoffman, manager of Research Technology Services. "People won't have to move all their data and research materials into the portal itself. By using the campus network infrastructure, they should be able to run their data locally but get it displayed in space." The unique campus has wide resources and facilitates collaboration across a wide range of disciplines, he notes. Visualization has been applied for years in fields such as physics, atmospheric sciences, chemistry and engineering. But recently it has become more multi disciplinary, as researchers in entertainment, the arts, humanities and health sciences have begun to put the technique to important uses. (Taubes, G., 2000) (www.ucla.edu/portal).

Molecular-scale computers hold the promise of putting the calculating ability of today's most powerful supercomputers in a chip the size of a grain of sand. In 1984, Jim Heath, a UCLA chemist and a graduate student, in the laboratory at Rice University, met Rick Smalley, a future Nobel laureate. Upon Day One, Jim Heath found himself confronted by a machine technically called a "laser-supersonic cluster beam apparatus" which Heath described more colorfully as "this huge, two-story contraption that had all sorts of lasers around it and no one to run it." Smalley, who designed the device (which was capable of vaporizing materials to study their constituent atoms or molecules), instructed Heath in the fine points of its operation and together they began to collect data.

This creation and discovery opened an entirely new branch of chemistry, led to the Nobel Prize in 1996 for Smalley and the other two senior collaborators, Bob Curl of Rice and Harry Kroto of the University of Sussex in England. It also sealed Heath's reputation as a graduate student and scientist of great promise. Heath's post doctoral fellow at UCLA as a resulted from his latest work—the creation of a futuristic computer architecture based on molecular switches and quantum wires so thin they are only several atoms across—appears in July (2000) on the front page of The New York Times under the headline "Tiniest Circuits Hold Prospect of Explosive Computer Speeds." Heath is now the principal investigator in a $8-million dollar endeavor, funded jointly by the Defense Advanced Research Project Agency and Hewlett-Packard Corporation, to turn these tiny circuits into a workable computer. (This integral research marks a turn in computers, making them more efficient, performing vast operations per second while consuming very little power.) Heath is also working on manufacturing technology of the future: a "bottom-up" manufacturing method of chemically assembling his molecular computers and other devices so small that millions could be fit on the head of a pin (Taubes, G., 2000).

The notion falls into the realm of nanotechnology, a discipline existing at the intersection of science fiction and science fact that is so exciting and promising that Business Week recently annoited it one of its 21 great ideas for the 21st century. (Literally, nano, form Greek nanos, or dwarf means 1-billionth part of, as in a nanosecond.) Indeed, in January, 2000, President Clinton announced his proposal to launch a $225-million, multiagency National Nanotechnology initiative, promising potential breakthroughs in everything from materials and manufacturing to medicine, agriculture, computation, the environment and national security (Hamilton, P., 2000).

Heath had convinced UCLA that computers and other such devices could be synthesized chemically—from the bottom up—rather than by etching the necessary circuits out of slabs of silicon, which is how chips are made today. He has generated a host of research projects based on this infinitesimal scale of chemistry. His work is on quantum dots, which Heath calls artificial atoms or nanoparticles, tiny chunks of perhaps a thousand atoms of a single element. Heath and his colleagues have made artificial solids out of these artificial atoms, and they have learned to precisely control the properties of these solids, turning them effortlessly from insulation to semiconductors to superconductors. There are all kinds of "gee-whiz things" one could do with such artificial solids, says Heath, his favorite being the synthesis of sensors that would react to day, a single photon of light by changing from an insulator to a semiconductor or even a superconductor. The promising molecular-sized computers are reaching barriers in speed and efficiency set by fundamental physical limits (Wilson, 1999). As silicon devices get smaller and smaller, they begin to edge into a realm in which quantum-mechanical effects become important. To pass this quantum-mechanical barrier requires devices that are inherently quantum mechanical, which is not the case with silicon semiconductors but it is with molecular switches. Heath calls the promise of molecular computers "fantastically amazing" and adds "it's very rare in any physical science that you see an operational improvement of a billion that's just waiting there to be tapped." Molecular-scale computers hold the promise of putting the calculating ability of today's most powerful supercomputers in a chip the size of a grain of sand. The potential applications are limited only by the power of the imagination (Taubes, G., 2000).

The Visible Human Project has launched a long-range planning effect of the National Library of Medicine (NLM) (O'Shaughnessy, K., 2000). As a result of this project, the long-range plan should "thoroughly and systematically investigate the technical requirements for and feasibility of instituting a biomedical images library. According to Dr. Michael J. Ackerman, Ph.D. (1994), the goal of this system of knowledge is to transparently link visual knowledge formats or structural informatics. The need for super computers goes on and on. The researchers all agree that tomorrow's medicine relies on today's resources. New technology is propelling into the future. Integration of computer systems to virtual reality is playing a strong role in planning programs used to improve patient diagnosis, treatment and long-term cure. Effective use of this technology will produce desired results according to researchers (Persico, 1997).

Moving forward in the midst of uncertain waters, hospitals are experiencing depressed revenue and ongoing expense control difficulties. Navigating the new millennium will need technology such as developed at Canadian hospitals. According to a news brief in <u>Advance For Administrators In Radiation Oncology</u>, October 1998, Vol. 8, Number 10, p. 15) (Blonshine, S., 1998), this could revolutionize brain surgery by cutting operating time in half and reducing hospital stays by 90 percent, say researchers. The technology-image-guided minimally invasive therapy (IGMIT) uses state-of-the-art magnetic resonance imagery (MRI) to provide surgeons with a real-time image of where they are operating and the precise location of instruments.

Before the technology became available, surgeons had to rely on MRI images taken before surgery. However, because the brain's geography is apt to change, those picture were not reliable. "IGMT allows surgeons to plan a more direct route to the target avoiding major structures and minimizing trauma, and to verify immediately after the operation whether it was successful or not," say Michael Bronskill, M.D., Director of Imaging, Bioengineering Research at Toronto's Sunnybrook Health Science Center. The technology is the result of a three-year, $22 million multi-disciplinary effort.

Intraoperative Computerized Tomography (CT) is vital for use with navigation systems because of the accuracy. Radiologists are heading back into the operating room (Tamas, 1997). The movement described by neurosurgeons at an international meeting held in Philadelphia recently discussed image-guided surgery and intraoperative computed tomography. These modalities are among the first of many emergency modalities that will change the face of radiology and surgery in the 21st Century (Ward, J., 1998).

The Stealth Platform integrates all digital imaging: Computerized Tomography (CT), Magnetic Resonance Image (MRI), Position Emission Tomography (PET), Single Photon Emission Computed Tomography (SPECT) and Ultrasound (US). With this image guidance system it allows surgeons to perform surgery effectively (Smith, K., 1994). Administrators calculate the saving on human resources for intraoperative imaging balance the competing needs of cost-efficiency, flexibility and imaging power.

Continued assumption is hospital health care is an expensive service that medical plans, Health Maintenance Organizations (HMO), and Pay Per Office (PPO) would make more money if the services performed were less extensive and more efficient (Goodman, G., 1997).

Working through transitions, reform, cost savings and accountable scientific methods, virtual imagery, new spacial reconstruction and implementation of artificial intelligences will meet the greater need than the past and present performances have experienced since the development of Computer Assisted Design (CAD) intelligence (Strauss, J., 1995).

OBJECTIVE OF STUDY

The purpose of this study is to assess, review, investigate advances in high technology medical systems for research and development of advanced medical diagnosis and treatment.

Interventions to promote futuristic space technologies require long range planning with financial support. Medical breakthroughs are ongoing. The monitoring of research and strong government backing will insure success in health care management (Strauss, J., 1995).

Research is a slow process. The high competitive market conducts research behind closed doors to contain confidentiality. Until patents are awarded companies regard research as secretive. Theoretically, classified information could compromise the legalistic outcomes. A planned technology acquisition strategy is crucial to survival (Smith, R., 1998).

The search for a successor to silicon has become a crusade; it is the Holy Grail of computation. Among physicists, the race to create the Silicon Valley for medical treatments for the next century has already begun. Some of the theoretical options are being explored (Van Winkle, 1998):

The optical computer: This computer replaces electricity with laser light beams. Unlike wires, light beams can pass through one another, making possible three-dimensional microprocessors. An optical transistor has already been invented; unfortunately, the components are still rather large and clumsy. The optical counterpart of a desktop computer would be the size of a car (Havanaugh-Brown, 1999).

The DNA computer: One of the most ingenious ideas being pursued is to compute using DNA, treating the double-stranded molecule as a biological computer tape (except that instead of encoding Os anls in binary, it uses the four nucleic acids, represented by A,T,C,G). This approach holds much promise for crunching big numbers. Hence large banks and institutions may one day use it. However, a DNA computer is an unwieldy contraption, consisting of a jungle of tubes of organic liquid, and is likely to replace the laptop in the near future (Kaker, 2000).

Molecular and Dot computers: Other exotic designs include the molecular computer and the quantum dot computer (which replace the silicon transistor with a single molecule and a single electron, respectively). But these approaches face formidable technical problems, such a mass-producing atomic wires and insulators. No viable proto types yet exist.

The Quantum computer: The dark horse to emerge from this race is the quantum computer, sometimes dubbed the ultimate computer. The idea is to direct a laser or radio beam on a carefully arranged collection of atomic nuclei, each of which is spinning like a top. As the beam bounces off the atoms, it flips and spins some of them. Complex computations can be performed by analyzing how the spins have been flipped (Quantum Teleportation, 1996).

QUANTUM COMPUTING

The U.S. Army is developing a quantum code machine that uses a form of tele-portation—recreating information at a distance (httpill.www.research.ibm.com/ quantum infor/teleportations/2000) to decode a message so that only one person can receive the message even when it is broadcast over open channels. The person on the receiving end gets a code based on quantum entanglement and decodes the message. This process is known as entanglement when, for example, electrons exist between two energy states. Normally, they have a discreet energy level. When in between, the two particles can be separated by a large distance and when one is affected the other reflects the same change in an apparent violation of a rule we have all been trained to believe. The quantum world is sort of a phantom world of half particles and half wave disappearing and reappearing in a discreet and digital fashion. At the lowest levels of particle physics, the world works more like a digital watch than an analog dial and face type.

In this sometimes ghostlike world of moving between states, some very complex relationships have been discovered that will allow quantum particles to be used like on and off bits of the computer except they have states. It was theorized that more qubits could be used to compute. The first quantum computers have done some very simple computations to demonstrate that the principle works. In fact, one of the first runs on caffeine molecules. The first simple structures have done simple calculations and other small steps toward testing quantum calcula-tions—they will not compete with the standard computers for years—but if it can be done in small scale, then researchers will generally find a way to do it on a large scale.

It has become imperative to study that quantum computation when the Shor algorithm (http://www-dse.doc.ic.ac.uk/-nd/surprise 97/journal/vol4/spb31) was developed by Peter Shor of Bell Laboratories. He posited that a quantum com-puter could factor a large number in seconds and render almost any secure com-puter transaction visible to the owner of such a computer. This fact caused NATO, the U.S. Military and other researchers to investigate the possibilities as soon as they could. Now it is no longer a question of if, but when this event will occur.

An algorithm developed by Lou Grover will sort an unsorted database faster than a conventional computer. The algorithm searches a multitude of universes with a single search and would theoretically crack the Data Encryption Standard (DES) that is used to protect things such as financial transactions between banks.

Add in the Army's "quantum beaming" communication device will send a code to another location that can only be detected by the person that is intended to receive it. The point of this existence, the average person would have no way of knowing about this work. The Web however has changed the way we think and work. Artificial intelligence may become a reality because a quantum computer theoretically can simulate any object.

Quantum communications happen faster than the speed of light. Some of quantum events may be happening in different dimensions or parallel universes. Entangled states of electrons when separated by distance, connect in a spooky way. When one is affected, the other is affected instantly. In order to imagine an explanation of other dimensions, assume we have a piece of paper and it has no thickness but has length and width. A two dimensional man living on this paper can move around within the limits of this "paper." From the outside we can watch him move freely from one corner to another and we can see both sides of the paper. We can stick out our finger into his 2D world and affect him. When one finger enters his world, he would see an object that looked like a circle. We would be a cross section of our finger that the plane of the 2D world crossed.

In our 3D world, you cannot imagine the next dimension. It is difficult to explain or predict the effects of the interaction of objects from other dimensions or parallel universes. Quantum particles or events appear to exist between these dimensions in some states and as we begin to build prediction models of their behavior. We try to model how they work. Researchers are finding that to predict their activities, you have to unbind yourself from the 3D universe.

Radiation is one form of quantum effects that researchers have all heard about and seen evidence of. None of this is completely new. Albert Einstein called this quantum mechanical correlation, a spooky action at a distance. You can find 116,000 documents on the subject quantum communications (2000).

Quantum Links: Quantum parallelism

http://www.doc.ic.ac.uk/-"ids/quantum-computing.html

Centre for Quantum Computation, University of Oxford:

http://www.qubit.org/

U.S. Army Research Office:

http://www.aro.army.mil/phys/roadmap.htm

U.S. intelligence agencies are nervously eyeing these new designs. Quantum computers, in particular, could be so powerful that they might one day break the most intricate secret codes the CIA can concoct. A quantum supercomputer is not going to leap out of some laboratory and paralyze the CIA anytime soon, because computers seem to be exquisitely sensitive. The tiniest disturbance—even a passing cosmic ray—can change the orientation of their computational atoms, spoiling the calculation. At present, quantum computers can perform only trivial calculations on perhaps five atoms. To do any useful work, they would need to calculate on millions of atoms. Evolution says organisms are replaced by species of superior adaptability. Self accelerating technologies make faster computers and may have a destabilizing effect on society.

In seeking to make a machine that passes the so called "turning test"—responses that would be indistinguishable from those of humans—artificial intelligence (AI) has proven to be a disappointment. The turning test may be an unfair measurement of AI process. "On Computational Wings: Rethinking the Goals of Artificial Intelligence," Kenneth M. Ford and Patrick J. Hayes maintain that the obsession with the turning test has led AI researchers down the wrong path. They drew an analogy with artificial flight. Engineers for centuries tried to produce flying machines by mimicking the way that birds soar, but modern aircraft obviously do not fly like birds, and fortunately so. From this argument, Ford and Hayes note that AI is effective in instrumentation and in data recognition tasks. "Expert" systems such as medical-diagnostic programs, search software, use intelligent agents, which roam cyberspace to retrieve information [see "intelligent Software" (Mases, P., 1995).

Several more AI projects exist. One is that of Douglas B. Lenat of Cycorp in Austin, Texas, who for more than a decade has been working on CYC, a project that aims to create a machine that can share and manage information, researchers consider this common sense [see "Artificial Intelligence," by Douglas B. Lenat, Scientific American, September 1995]. Rodney Brooks and Lynn Andrea Stein of the Massachusetts Institute of Technology, whose team has produced Cog, a humanoid robot that its makers hope to endow with abilities of a conscious human, without its necessarily being conscious. AI sparks feelings of anxiety. Game-playing machines ("Computers, Games and the Real World," Gingsberg, 1995), Matthew L. Ginsberg summarizes the contests machines are playing and how they fare against human competitions. Gary Kasparov's loss in a six-game match against IBM's Deep Blue last year may have inspired some soul searching. The point of game-playing computers is not so much to best their makers as to explore which types of calculations are best suited to the architecture of the silicon chip. As Ginsberg reminds us, computers are designed not to replace humans but to help us. Life with computers is intelligence. Alex P. Pentland (1995) explains how devices such as keyboards, monitor screens, wireless transmitters and receivers are getting so small that we can physically wear them. Imagine reading e-mail on special glasses as you walk down the street, generating power in your shoes that converts to electricity which powers your persona-area network for cellular communications. Two M.I.T. students, Thad Starner and Steve Mann, have spent time in such cyborg existences—Stearner, 1992. A true melding of mind and machine is still far away, but the appeal is irresistible.

British Telecommunications has a project called Soul Catcher; the goal is to develop a computer that can be slipped into the brain to augment memory and other cognitive functions. Hans Moravec of Carnegie Mellon University and other researchers have argued, somewhat disturbingly, that it should be possible to remove the brain and download its contents into a computer—and with it, one hopes, personality and consciousness. Connecting neurons to silicon is only in its infancy. Peter Fromherz and his colleagues at the Max Planck Institute of Biochemistry in Martinsried-Munchen, Germany, have managed to connect the brain with a computer chip and caused the neuron to fire when instructed by the computer chip. Granting that neuron used in the experiment came from a leech, sets pace for interdiscipline studies in biology and biochemical research to help create intelligent computer systems. Expert systems, notes co-organizer Eric Horvitz of Microsoft Research, do quite well in their singular tasks but cannot match an invertebrate in behavior flexibility. If researchers knew what a synapse was doing they could mimic it. The hydrocarbon basis of neurons might also mean that the brain is more efficient with its constituent materials than a computer is with its silicon. Researchers do not have the mathematical foundation yet states Chris Dione of the University of Washington (Ford, Kant, Hayes, 2000).

EXPECTED RESULTS

Exploitation of advanced technologic systems "A Look to the Future" provides information regarding surgical, medical diagnosis and treatment centers via Web, 2000 E Commerce medical practices (Weber, T., 2000).

The Web is accelerating and improving the testing of new medical treatments according to Fred Sandsmark, California Computer New, September 2000. Clinical trials are run by strict rules set by the U.S. Food and Drug Administration (FDA). Clinical trials involve many years, millions of dollars for diagnosis, testing and evaluating new treatments, new drugs and cost concerns. Using quantum physics, medical doctors, biochemist engineers in interdiscipline labs, examine the applications in medicine for better health care delivery. The acceleration of research and development technology, a study-data phase, is accelerated on Phase Forward (<http://www.phaseforward.com.), by a Waltham mass-based company that's developing clinical trial data collection, management software and services. As more and more clinical trial processes are handled online, new ways to improve the system will emerge. The goal researchers is to "open the pipeline for better, faster development of new and better medical treatment.

Treatment with drug therapy: "The only reason you're able to take a drug is because its been through a clinical trial." explained David Restrepo, Vice President for business development at Acurian, a company that's developing Internet tools for the clinical trials process. The Pharmaceutical Researchers and Manufacturers Association (PhRMA) reports 369 biotechnology medicines are currently in development—up from 143 just seven years ago. To sell these new drugs, researcher companies need clinical trials. Many clinical trials are called "multicenter trials." This meas that many doctors test one treatment all over the country. (Doctors who assist with the clinical trials are referred to as "investigators.") A multicenter trial has many advantages: it gets more diverse groups of patients in the test pool, it distributes the work of recruiting patients, it collects data, and it tests the treatment on many people simultaneously. To streamline the recruiting process Acurian has built a website called Aculaunch (<http;//www. aculanch.coma.) Aculaunch allows pharmaceutical companies to search through Acurian's proprietary database of nearly 50,000 physicians who have been active as clinical investigators. Funding patients to participate in clinical trials has never been easy. Investigators usually resort to "searchlight" approach—putting out messages by mass media T.V. ads, phone drives, newspaper ads, and radio time. With the advent of website for specific diseases, the patient comes to them. The FDA is helping with a clinical trial information website {<http://www. clinicaltrials.gov.); it provides explanations of diseases in layman's language. Once patients have been recruited for a clinical trial, the record keeping process begins.

Chapter 2, Review of Literature provided a comprehensive assessment of studies reported on virtual reality in medicine, supported by studies and reported characteristics of trends in hospital health delivery.

Specific attention is given to artificial aided diagnosis, integration of MRI, CT, PET, SPECT and digital radiology, and Internet surgical-aided smart brain centers with artificial intelligence.

Chapter 3, Conclusion and Recommendations, epitomized the facts to summarize hospital investment and procurement of monies for technological delivery systems. As managed care becomes more widely distributed throughout the country, health care plans want medical services based on cost, quality, customer satisfaction, and positive outcomes. The competitive edge for mega-hospital corporations is to rely on the ability to acquire these new systems, implement training, engage physician participation and fuse information in both anatomy, function of anatomy and delivery treatment. Volume rendering and 3-D reconstruction techniques create virtual images, "fly through" hollow grams of organs, using endoscopy procedures to reduce radical medical treatment, quicker diagnosis, and cost less than today's common medical practices—a doorway to alternative medicine practices.

2

REVIEW OF RELATED LITERATURE

In the last decade computers have seeped into every aspect of our lives. The evolution of the computer has been and will continue to be a phenomenal example of problem solving ingenuity. Computers have come a long way from the first adding machine, devised in 1642 by the French philosophy and mathematician Blaise Pascal.

In 1993, the first meeting held in San Diego, California:

MEDICINE MEETS

VIRTUAL REALITY I

Interactive technology and health care. Visionary applications for simulation… Visualization…Robots.

The University of California, San Diego School of Medicine, has focused on the health care applications of virtual reality technologies. Simulation, visualization, and robotics—are leading edge technologies in the future of medical and surgical practice. This forum was a unique method to interact with researchers, to alter the way health care provides exchange of information, and methods for improving access, quality and of medical procedures while reducing cost for better medical outcomes.

- <u>Biological Informatics</u>. Science has benefited from technology's computer driven advances that help to create and store a cornucopia of raw data and information. As a result of data-overcrowding, it has become increasingly difficult to identify hypothesis that can be used to guide experimental and clinical research.

- <u>Massively Parallel Processing Computers for Medical Technology Development</u>. Is used for creating an efficient medical data base, creating a fast, powerful simulation approach, and analyzing complicated signals images in an economic way. Massively Parallel Processing (MPP) computers are becoming very attractive to develop new technology in medical fields.

- Interactive Technologies in Health Care: The Big Picture. The overall view of emerging human-computer interface.

A. MEDICAL AND VIRTUAL REALITY

With all its advantages, computer visualization technologies still imply a separation between the user and technology. For instance, a person may enhance their knowledge through three-dimensional imaging, but researchers are still on the outside looking in. Researchers are one step removed from the data base, the same way a television viewer is involved in a given program, is ultimately watching the program, not participating.

However, virtual reality (VR) is changing the very definition of the media experience. The term virtual reality refers to techniques that represent the ultimate application of computer technology. VR is so-called because it places the participant right in the middle of a computer-created environment. To date, it represents the closest thing to a final merging of cybernetic techniques and human experience, involving the participant in a visual and tactile experience that borders real life.

In 1986, science/science fiction writer William Gibson in a novel called Neuromancer, introduced a concept called cyberspace, a region existing in the world of information that researchers can visit but not touch (corporate data banks, computer conferrencing systems, and books). In a sense, every time a researcher calls a data bank, turns on the computer to browse a file, or plays a videogram, the researcher has entered into cyberspace. There is a vast difference between experiencing the information images in cyberspace on a computer screen in VR. VR, according to cybernauts who use such systems, are directly in the vision (Dumay, 1994).

This near real experience is accomplished with the aid of highly sophisticated technology. The Eye Phone is a bulky set of goggles that the cybernaut places on his head. These goggles project images directly onto the eye. The user looks through these goggles and watches lifelike images that seem to be part of his field of vision. The goggles are connected to the head with sensors, so that as the wearer turns his head, the field of vision changes. He imagines that he is spanning the horizon.

The Dataglove, which is fitted to the hand and enables the hand to become part of the computer's simulated field of vision, aids the viewer to allow manipulation of objects in VR—rearranging furniture, mountain tops, human anatomy, data bank information, etc. (Greenleaf, W., 1994).

The best application of VR apparatus allows one to "walk through" the artificial images in cyberspace. It allows researchers to simulate a structure in the environment, and "see" just where the researchers went wrong before the structure has been assembled. VR takes computer visualization to its conceptual limits. It allows not only visual reality but also a quantitative or mathematically representation of reality.

One intriguing application of VR to the field of medicine is currently being tested at the University of North Carolina at Chapel Hill. Here, a physician wearing VR headgear can see ultrasound images as he looks at the uterus of a woman lying in front of him. Video cameras are placed on both sides of his headgear so that the ultrasound images of the fetus are superimposed on his external view. The physician sees through the patient. According to Gary Bishop, a research associate professor at the university, the doctor "can see thorough a three-dimensional position of a baby in the mother's body." Such precision may make VR a perfect tool for brain surgery. Bishop claims that a VR-assisted neurosurgeon "holds the probe, sees the tumor underneath and knows the angle to enter" (Durlach, N., 1994).

The implications of VR's role in the expansion of human potential may transcend the linkage with biofeedback. A researcher at Wright-Patterson Air Force Base has developed an apparatus that allows the participant to play a flight simulation videogram without manipulating the hand and finger but by changing brain wave lengths. Captain David Tumey has set a system up in such a way that a flight video simulator can pilot an aircraft from another aircraft. The subject uses not hand-held mouse or joystick, but uses his own brain waves.

VR forum—interfaces medicine to create the future of medical treatment and health care. Connect (the weekly newsletter of UCSD Connect 2000) is an example of tomorrow's leading edge in technology. Connect Forum recognizes the need for dissemination of ideas and information related to emerging techniques in medical treatments. A multi-specialty, interdisciplinary forum includes health care providers, researchers, and developers of technology in utilizing hospitals. When services are rendered, the assumption is that hospital health care providers are expensive, increasing patient barriers, limiting surgical procedures, delaying diagnosis, using cheaper drug therapy and insisting on shorter hospital stays or possibly refuse expensive treatment entirely. Working through transitions, reform, cost savings and accountable scientific methods will bring to forefront new spacial reconstruction implementation of artificial intelligence. When the need is greater than past performance, change will occur.

The surgical options for brain tumors are determined by the best method of treatment for each patient. New developments in computed tomography (CT) scanning are positioning the modality to play a strong role in image-guided surgery. During the coming years, new, expanded diagnostic, interventional applications of CT angiography, CT fluoroscopy, hepatic imaging techniques and cardiovascular applications will be the standard in medical treatment and diagnosis, according to Joyce Ward, CNMT(N) (1998).

Images from CT can be fused with scans from functional magnetic resonance imaging (MRI), positron emission tomography (PET) or single photon emission computed tomography (SPECT) to provide physicians with information on both the anatomy and function. New instrumentation allows radiologic technologies to take thinner slices in less time, improving multi planar and 3-D images.

With the minimally invasive surgical devices, imaging equipment is increasingly being used in surgical planning evaluation and procedures. Imagery-guided surgery is used in planning approaches to brain, head and neck surgery, indicated Fereca Jolesz, M.D., Professor of Radiology at Harvard Medical School and director of the image-guided therapy program at Brigham and Woman's Hospital, Boston (Ward, J, 1998). Radiologists are headed to the OR. (Medical historians cite 1904 when neurosurgeon Anton von Eisenberger joined neurologist Otto Mabenburg and the world-famous neuro-anatomist Julius Tandler, who directed the surgeon to the tumor with a radiograph.)

In the last decade, computers have seeped into every aspect of American life. They are used for everything from constructing models of the universe to withdrawing spending money from the local bank. The evolution of the computer has been, and continues to be, a phenomenal example of problem solving and ingenuity. The field of medicine, specifically radiology, has not been exempt from this computer explosion (Steven, P. 1997).

Digital devices are playing an increasing role in how radiology personnel perform their tasks. The necessity of timely sharing patient information with departments in the hospital has administrators taking a hard look at how computers may solve many problems hospitals face. Manufacturers recognize little is to be gained by keeping proprietary image format. Efforts were made to standardize radiology information. A committee was formed by the American College of Radiology (ACR) in collaboration with the National Electrical Manufacturers Association. Their objective was to develop an interface so that images and related information could be exchanged between medical imaging equipment and an interface. The committee developed an interface called the DICOM, or digital imaging and communication in medicine.

DICOM was designed with three main purposes: 1) promote communications of digital image information regardless of device or manufacturer, 2) facilitate the expansion of PACS that can also interface with other systems of hospital information, and 3) allow the creation of diagnostic information databases that can be examined by a wide variety of devices and distributed geographically (Steven, P., 1997).

One of the first objectives of a Picture Archives Communication System (PACS) is to collect radiologic images in digital form for storage and future viewing. A computerized patient record must be complete and able to handle multimedia data from different sources. Although there is a significant percentile of radiologic images that are collected directly in digital form, such as CT and MRI, manufacturers have historically been reluctant to provide an easy way to access the images (Schilling, R., 1995).

In the past, PACS had to deal with serious difficulties in extracting the images from the many different types and brands of acquisition devices. Expensive customized interfaces had to be developed by a programmer that could create an application that addressed the needs of a specific organization. Also, manufacturing had to be persuaded into releasing often proprietary information.

Other standards have also been developed to help integrate PACS with other relevant information. The HL7, or health level seven, attempts to standardize integration information system implementations. The digital interchange standard for cardiology or DISC, extends DICOM to cardiology applications (Stevens, P., 1997).

These applications to medicine have allowed transfer information to be used on workstations as The Stealth Platform. (Smith, B., 1997) New and extensive research is actively joining medical professionals. The Stealth Platform will change the way surgical components are applied to treatment of tumors, diseases and conditions (Smith, K., 1994).

Hard-dollar justifications are difficult as a means to purchase PACS. Indeed, it must be considered that PACS will play a key role in the development of an information network infrastructure that is critical to the long-term profitability of the facility (Roman, L., 1997).

In most hospitals the balance of power in the decision-making process has shifted from department based decisions to a team approach. Although radiology is a critical component in the team, it is often anchored by information systems, communications, and other internal and external information resources. When surveyed, radiology administrators significantly underestimated the cost of their image management system. Radiology consultants and researchers have estimated that the cost of a nondigital film management can exceed $2 million dollars annually per 100,000 procedures. This figure can be broken down as follows: 20 percent film, 35 percent technologist and clerical labor (overhead), 20 percent referring physician time, and 25 percent radiologist time.

The different mechanisms exist for connecting computers to peripheral devices. Hard drives can vary with the time it takes to read an image on the disk, decompress the image, and display it on the computer screen. This is referred to as the disk access time and is measured in milliseconds. Disk access time is important to the perception of work station performance particularly with the large radiographic image files.

Different mechanisms exist for connecting computers to peripheral devices, such as hard disk and prints, and they greatly influence access speed. In general, the fastest and preferred method is the SCSI (pronounced Scuzzy), which is an acronym for small computer system interface. Up to seven devices, not including this computer can be attached through a single SCSI connection. ASCSI is also used to connect a computer to other computers and a local area network (LAN).

It is to be expected that the greatest impact of this technology will not occur in radiology, but will have a substantial effect on referring physicians, nurses, and other health care practitioners, managing the medical care utilizing personnel, and finally, patients.

For this reason, the perception of a PACS outside of radiology has undergone a major change in the past few years. PACS are no longer seen as radiology's solution to a problem that only impacts radiology. Instead, they are viewed as playing an essential role in an integrated hospital-wide information and image management solution.

Images that are already digitized are relatively easy to include in a PACS. Hospitals often start with ultrasound and incrementally add CT, MRI and nuclear medicine. These networks are called modality clusters or mini-PACS. Some imaging centers have instituted modality cluster PACS and have received a return on the initial investment in less than a year. An imaging department with one CT and one ultrasound unit performing ten cases per modality per day, can save nearly $30,000 in film costs a year by using an optical archive to save images (Romans, L., 1997).

When implementing a mini-PACS it is important to look to the future and plan how (and if) it will be integrated into a complete PACS. For example, archiving on CD Rom works well for a modality cluster, but not as well for a complete PACS, where digital tape for archiving is likely to be a better choice.

Few hospitals can afford to implement an entire PACS in a single fiscal year. Instead, a step-by-step approach is common. Not only can the cost of the system be spread out but phasing in a PACS can help to reduce the culture shock to the hospital staff. Many physicians and technologists have trouble adjusting to the new digital management systems. Changing their attitude toward the new technology can be a major hurdle and must be addressed in the implementation strategy. Suddenly elementary hard copy film can result in a huge disruption to all hospital operations.

The ability of a work station to interact with other work stations is referred to as networking. A local area network is a group of computers connected by cables or wireless communication that share applications, data, and peripherals (such as printers). A LAN does not use telephone lines, so it is typically contained within a single building or campus. Usually a LAN is wired through a "hub" so any work station can access another work station via the network. Work stations that are hard-wired together in this manner are usually faster than those that receive shared data over a phone line or other communications line.

The wire that is used to connect the work stations in a LAN is called a media. Different classes of media are available and will affect the speed of data transmission.

A system that connects computers to others that are geographically distance is called a WAN, or wide area network. This system uses some form of telecommunication, and the information sent is generally slower than that sent over a LAN.

Different methods of attaching work stations to computers are greatly influenced by the medical professionals systems like the Stealth Work Station performing integrated applications for surgical procedures. The contribution for future non-invasive surgical procedures rely on advanced technology. In this situation, the Stealth Work Station demands multiple expertise in radiology and a skilled surgeon to perform these new treatments (Smith, B., 1997).

B. Stealth Station Improves Doctor's Surgical Visions

The "stealth economy" in Colorado is top-secret radar and high-tech communications system but there is another aspect to the state's "stealth" industry in the medical field. The technology is called the "Stealth Station" and it is designed for the inner space of the human body. Using a medical computer work station, Stealth Station helps surgeons pinpoint such things as brain tumors (Kormos, D., 1994).

Dr. Stewart Levy, a neurosurgeon at St. Anthony Hospital Central, said the technology enables the surgeon to precisely map out the margins of a brain tumor that otherwise might be invisible to the eye. Physicians have used such things as MRI and CT scans to locate a tumor, but the Stealth Station translates those images into a tool that can be used during surgery. The technology displays the MRI and CT scans as a "global reference" to the patient's skull, giving the surgeon real-time visualization of the location of his operative instruments (Smith, B., 1997).

> "The reason it is so important is that a lot of brain tumors are not that much different [visually from normal brain matter]," said Levy, "When you're in the operating room with the patient's head open, you can't tell where the tumor is. But it shows up on the MRI and you can map out the margins of the tumor based on the imaging and delineate exactly where it is. You won't damage the normal brain, but can completely remove the tumor. It decreases the risks to the patient; it reduces the risk of paralysis."

St. Anthony Central, which bought one of the $350,000 units last fall, is one of 73 hospitals world-wide using the Stealth technology. Another Colorado based tie to the Stealth Station. The software development and system integration was engineered by a Broomfield Company of Colorado.

Surgical Navigation Technology, Inc. (SNT, 1997) was a privately held company until its acquisition in April 1996 by one of the nation's leading medical device companies, Sofamor Danek Group, Inc. Of Memphis, Tennessee. Stealth Station did not clear FDA approval until 1996, but now is selling eight a month. The technology currently is used for cranial, spinal, ear-nose-throat and radio surgeries, with potential future applications in orthopedics and even cancer biopsies, according to Kurt Smith, SNT's founder and chief technical officer.

C. Silicon Graphics Oxygen Computer

The technologies exist that provide 3-D visualization of anatomical features with real $\pm$ cm. localization information. With Stealth Platform, the physician takes standard image data sets from most image sources and transforms them into three dimensional volumes, utilizing a sophisticated silicon graphics O2 computer.

This is how it works. When the surgeon's instrument touches the patient's anatomy, an optical scanner mounted above the operating table locates the instrument and establishes a 3-D location. The instrument location is entered from the operative filed through the digitizer to the silicon graphics O2 computer. The 02 computer registers, or matches, the anatomy to the patient's preoperative C.T. or MR data. The powerful graphical and computing abilities of the O2 indicate the instrument's location on a high resolution monitor proximate to the surgeon's location in the operating room. Lines depicting the instrument's position are displayed over the patient's MR scans.

The physician can following in real-time the precise location of the surgical instruments such as: bipolar forceps, admit guide, an endoscope, or a microscope focal point within the body. This technology is referred to as computer assisted or image-guided surgery. There has been more than 4,500 surgical cases performed on SNT.

The United States and other countries will be able to expand that knowledge quickly through research (Human Genome Project, Stephenson, J., 1998). Through the use of computer programs such as Cal Tech's genetic sequencer, researchers have cataloged the 100,000 or so genes that direct the makings of proteins in the body. The explanation for expansion of genetic research enables the medical professional to predict an individual's propensity for disease, even at the fetal stage.

According to geneticist Michael Hayden of the University of British Columbia, "We're looking at a totally new form of medicine, preventive medicine." According to Hayden, the new hope is that we can employ a gene first to predict the risk of a disease and then to modify the genetic make up to prevent the disorder.

Through gene mapping a number of disease-related genes already have been identified: 1. Fragile X mental retardation, 2. Muscular dystrophy, 3. Hemophilia, 4. Cystic fibrosis, 5. Sickle-cell anemia, 6. Breast cancer, 7. Eye cancer, 8. Colon cancer, and 9. Coronary atherosclerosis (Hayden, M., 1998).

Gene therapy will transcend genetic mapping and diagnosis. In 1990 an NIH team led by Michael Blaise performed the first successful treatment of the "bubble-boy disease" which is a genetic condition lacking a functioning immune system. This disease which afflicts children because they lack a specific enzyme (ADA), could be cured if the right gene for the enzyme was added to their blood cells. The team extracted the T-cells (from the immune system) and inserted normal ADA, helping the immune system to function effectively. After a few weeks the patients returned to the NIH for further successful treatment.

Pioneer Michael Blaise has tested a new treatment for severe combined immunodeficiency (SCID). He has inserted ADA into the "stem-cells" after a genetically engineered process to give rise to new blood cells. Now these patients are assured to produce a permanent supply of this enzyme.

Be sure that the best of possible worlds exist, particularly gene amplification. Cetus Corporation is a pioneer in developing a sleuth technology known as PCR—polymerase chain reaction. With this technology, technicians can locate and identify specific genes much more quickly and precisely than using other methods and hence identify the bacteria, virus, and mutant genes that cause disease.

The diagnostic revolution is further augmented by breakthroughs in fiber optics. These new technologies allow an internal view of anatomy, analyze blood using sensors and performs surgery with safe laser systems. The modern fiberscope is uniquely adapted to its mission. It consists of two bundles of optical fibers. Once, the illuminating bundle carries light to the tissues, and the other, called the imaging bundle, transmits the image to the observer.

New sensors have been developed that can analyze blood chemistry by measuring the hue and florescence of various biomolecules, making it possible to determine the blood's oxygen content directly. By studying the colors reflected inside various organs, detection of a patient's blood has the capacity to supply sufficient oxygen to his or her heart and lungs for these organs to function. This tool represents progress. It clearly enhances the ability of physicians and technologists to peer into the inner most parts of the human body. This also represents a noninvasive technique for exploring the body. The patient is spared the medical risks involved in old-style incisions and cutting. Diagnosis can be done without performing surgery.

The net effect of gene amplification fiber optics and long-distance diagnosis are profound. We no longer need experts in a particular pathology (e.g., blood disease) clustered in one location. Doctors in remote regions can perform fiber optic explorations and even show experts from different facilities results via satellite. Video conferencing is not an unlikely derivative of this technology—several conferencing simultaneously perhaps even controlling through joysticks, the fiberscope's journey through a patient's intestines. Super drug designers are investing millions of dollars to fight a myriad of diseases. These new super drugs are synthetics and relatively inexpensive to manufacture. A process called pharming is a better method for developing human hormones or proteins than the use of bacterial cultures. Companies are utilizing what is known as "pharming" to alter relatives of common breeds of cattle, sheep, and goats genetically in order to endow such livestock with human genes. These genes enable transgenic animals to produce human hormones or proteins in large quantities. The process has led some scientists to label this animal bioreators.

The first step in pharming is to isolate the human gene for a desired protein (the Human Genome Project is making gene identification possible). The a string of genetic materials must be engineered that tells the host when and where to make the protein. Then we must selectively breed these transgenic males and females that produce the desired protein (Lau, E., 2000).

D. THE HUMAN GENOME PROJECT

The Goal:

The goal of the Human Genome Project was to generate a series of tools that will change the way biological research is carried out (Hayden, M., 1998). Much of the information required by a cell is stored in the nucleus, encoded into the structure of the DNA molecules that are called chromosomes. This information allows the cell to replicate, differentiate into all the different cells that comprise a human, interact with other cells, respond to that, replace damaged tissue, etc. An understanding of this information stored in the chromosomes would give biologists an insight into how the cell functions that would greatly accelerate information stored in the chromosomal DNA. This part of the project is known as DNA sequencing. There are 3 billion residues, or bases, in the human genome and it is in the order of these bases that encodes the biological information.

Other biological spinoffs occur along the way. Most of the chromosomes in a population are different; they differ at a rate of about 0.1%. Among these differences researchers look to find genes for diseases that act as an inherited component. This field of research is called genetics, and with the advent of the Genome Project, is becoming a powerful tool which enables biologists to decipher the reason behind many more common diseases that affect man. The basic tool is genetic maps. These are the road maps to the human genome using small pieces of DNA that are likely to differ between chromosomes.

In order to sequence the human genome, maps of the chromosomes based on the DNA of the chromosomes must be constructed. These maps are known as physical maps. The end product of a physical map is a series of overlapping pieces of DNA that have been isolated in bacteria. These pieces of DNA are ordered in the same order that they would appear in the human genome and are used as the templates for the sequencing project.

Obviously the information that comes from the Human Genome Project will have many ramifications for humankind. Changes in the sequences of the DNA that predisposes to diseases are being found almost daily. These will effect how insurance companies have access to information. A DNA fingerprint is more accurate than a real finger print in identifying an individual.

The race is over (Golden, F. & Lemonick, M., 2000). The great genome quest is official a tie. J. Craig Venter and Dr. Francis Collins are celebrating the completion of a project that will ultimately transform medicine more than vaccines and antibiotics combined. Dr. Francis Collins, director of the National Institute of Health, is the National Human Genome Research Institute project's unofficial head, and J. Craig Venter, CEO of Celera Genomics, an independent genome-sequencing project head, are trying to settle differences over who should get credit for completion of the genome sequence milestone.

Aristides (Ari) Patrinos, a scientist at the Department of Energy who directs the agency's share of the Human Genome Project, has been lobbying Dr. Collins and J. Craig Venter to put away their longstanding feud over differences in each researcher's scientific discovery. After a joint declaration by Clinton and British Prime Minister Tony Blair in March, 2000, that all genomic information should be free, the value of Celera stock plunged from $189 a share to $149.25.

After more than a decade of dreaming, planning and heroic number crunching, both groups have deciphered essentially all the 3.1 billion biochemical "letters" of human DNA, the code for building and operating a fully functional human. It is impossible to overstate the significance of this achievement. Armed with genic coding, scientists can now start selecting the secrets of human health and disease at the molecular level—secrets that will lead to revolution in diagnosing and treatment of Alzheimer's disease, to heart disease, transforming the start of the genome era.

While the announcement was to make the two scientists look like equals, its clear to the insiders that Venter's project is a lot further along. HGP scientists may have decoded 97% of the genomes letters—the remaining 3% are generally considered unsequenciable and irrelevant—but they know the order of only 53% of them. It's as if they've got the pages in the so-called book of life in the proper order but with the letters on each page scrambled.

Celera, by contrast, has not only the pages but all the words and letters as well. HGP boasts that it has gone over its sequence nearly seven times to guarantee accuracy. Celera has gone over its own sequence five times. The Celera company came up with a new technique that has made sequencing rate the fastest around. Venter claims that by the end of this year they will have sequenced the genome of a mouse—whose 2.3 billion letters contain enough similarities to ours to make it vitally important to scientists tracking down human gene function. Celera's analyses was done by robot gene sequencers and high-speed computers. Venter has declared his intention to sequence the entire human genome in only a fraction of time (three years) and at a much lower cost ($200 million) than government-sponsored scientists had originally said it would take: 15 years and $3 billion dollars. Venter lifted data made public on the government's GenBank website (www.nebi.^/m.gov) at taxpayer's expense and then patenting sequences called from this data, therefore locking up information originally intended to be freely available. (Ironically, Celera suffered a setback when some of the government data turned out to be contaminated with non-human sequences.)

Venter learned in 1986 about a machine that could "read" genes by shining lasers on their dyed letters (A,T,C, and G, the four nitrogenous bases—adenine, thymine, cytosine and guanine—that spells out the genome's "words"). He immediately went to meet its builder, Michael Hunkapiller in Foster City, California. This phototype helped Venter to decode 100,000 letters (the human genome has some 3.1 billion spelling out some 50,000 different genes at the best guess. They were hieroglyphics to him, but to living cells which recognizes active genes and spin off single strands of RNA that mirror the DNA's coding. So Venter collected the new RNA, inserting it into bacterial cells and letting them clone junk-free complimentary DNA or CDNA, matching the original genes. His automatic sequencer could read them and the letters of these genetic instructions.

In 1998, when Hunkapiller showed Venter his new ABI Prisom 3,700, a Sequencer five times as fast and more highly automated, Venter formed a partnership with Hunkapiller's company, Applied Biosystems (now PE Biosystems). Venter named his new outfit Celera, from the Latin word for "quick." It was backed with an infusion of $300 million from his new collaborator. Venter boldly announced that he would sequence and assemble the entire genome by the year 2001.

Venter says he'll be offering sophisticated, contamination-free, gift-edged data for comparison genomes of other species and genetics of specific diseases, plus special proprietary software to analyze this genetic mother code. Having signed up five major pharmaceutical houses as well as Vanderbuilt University, Venter says its company has jumped ahead of its rivals, with revenue doubling every year. Venter also plans to go through six more genomes, including his own. After the mouse, he plans on going through the chimp among our closest primate kin, and explore the plant genes, including rice and cord. Venter is taking Celera into the emerging field of proteomics—understanding how genes make and manage proteins, the actual building blocks of life.

Venter and Collins will never be collaborators given their dramatic differences. The two teams will try to publish their work simultaneously—but not jointly.

Mapping the genome is a highly complex process. Scientists at drug firms, biotech companies and university labs have taken literally hundreds of baby steps into the era of genomics medicine using an impressive array of powerful new tools. DNA chips and microarrays that let scientists see at a glance which of the thousands of genes are active in a given tissue sample. Sophisticated software can organize gigabytes of genetic data, and can organize huge data bases of genes, disease tissue samples and mRNA—the molecules that initiate the actual construction of working proteins. Understanding how and when genes make proteins will give doctors new ways of looking at disease and lead to new treatments (Golden, F. & Lemonick, M., 2000).

This data is supported by Digital DNA; A Smart Card developed by Motorola, which stores your insurance and medical information on a chip (www. dighita/dna.com, 2000).

E. VIRTUAL REALITY MEETS MEDICINE PROGRAM SUMMARY

Dr. George Poste, Chief Science & Technology Officer for Smith Kline Beacham, had a compelling overview of current issues in health care and the new tools biotechnology is sure to create. Through analysis of population genetics, customization of pharmaceuticals in clinical care will become a common tool in diagnoses, treatments, and even prevention in ways now impossible. The larger ramifications of a healthy world were explored by Dr. Poste (Next Med, 1998).

Research of Dr. Gregory Kovacs, Stanford University, in nanotechnologies (now micromachines) are transforming our ability to go into the body to diagnose and treat its ailments. Dr. Ted Berger of USC's Center for Neural Engineering discussed his research on microchips implanted in the brain and the likelihood of a hybrid organic silicon human brain, once science fiction, perhaps tomorrow's reality. One of the century's great theoreticians on the human brain, Dr. Karl Pribram, gave insights on his current work and new understanding of how our brain actually operates. Dr. Christopher Chernick of the University of

Maryland showed his findings on neural structure that revealed patterns of efficiency like those found in fluid mechanics.

Dr. Robert Strausberg and Dr. Carol Dahl of the National Cancer Institute discussed their research in cancer therapy and possibilities for greater specificity in clinical care based on information from the Human Genome Project. Dr. David Marshak of Osiris Therapeutics detailed his company's success using mesenchymal stem cells to regenerate tissue for damaged and degenerating body parts (Next Med, 1998).

Dr. Stephen Johnston of the University of Texas, Southwestern Medical Center, discussed his lab's work at the leading edge of genetic manipulation and tools that could be derived from new biological structures "created from scratch." Dr. Donald Ingber of the Harvard Medical School and Molecular Geodesics discussed his work in tissue engineering and manipulation of protein structure to create novel tools and treatments. Dr. Ronald Taylor of the University of Virginia explained his success in clearing pathogens from the blood stream by binding them with heteropolymers. Monsanto Company is said to form a broad technological alliance with IBM, focusing on genomics. Genomics can be used for everything from isolating a gene that causes or prevents diseases to developing plants that yield healing oils. The scientists from the two companies use Teiresias, an algorithm recently developed by IBM to detect hidden patterns in genes. The cornerstone of this alliance is a joint effort to map the genetic makeup of plant and human diseases.

Researchers at U.C. Davis Cancer Center have received grants totaling more than $1 million to study prostate cancer, the most common cancer affecting American men. Two projects investigating mutations of a tumor suppressor or gene that plays a major role in prostate cancer were awarded a total $605,000 from the National Cancer Institute and the federal Department of Defense to learn how alterations of a gene causes prostrate cancer. Another $424,393 from the Department of Defense was awarded to researchers for a way to treat more effectively patients' resistant to testosterone-blocking drugs. This year an estimated 330,000 men will be diagnosed with prostrate cancer and more than 40,000 will die from it (Next Med, 1998).

F. TIERRA: SUGARSCAPE SECRETS

Working from a model that gene code is analogous to computer code, several groups are working to create life from the bare savannah of silicon. One of the first and most recognized was the "Sugarscape" program developed by Joshu M. Epstein and John Axtell (1996) at the Brookings Institution in Washington, D.C.

As Epstein and Axtell reported in Science News (November 23, 1996), Sugarscape is a virtual world, a two-dimensional grid inhabited by basic software "agents" and certain resources which the agents need to survive. In the simplest form, there are two areas high in "sugar" resource, which can grow back after being consumed. Agents search as far as "vision permits, to find the unoccupied spot with the most sugar, go there, and eat the sugar" (basic hunter-gatherer philosophy).

Interestingly, recognizable trends begin to form when population rises, a minority of agents with better vision and lower metabolisms accumulate most of the sugar. The less fortunate majority often subsists in the sugar scrublands. Some die of starvation.

More significantly, when reproduction, mutation and inheritance of sugar resources are added, the foundations of a weak upper class are formed. Agents who might have been "weeded out" are given an extra advantage through inheritance.

Revelations continue to occur when a second resource, "spice," is added in conjunction with trade between tribes, a perfect economic equilibrium emerges as long as agents are immortal. Sugarscape economic model never reaches equilibrium. The implications for human economic theory are limited in view extrapolating a minuscule gene changes which fuel a species-wide metamorphosis takes tens of thousands, sometimes millions of years to become noticeable (Epstein, J., Axtell, J., 1996).

Enter artificial life, or "alife." Working from the model that gene code is analogous to computer code, several groups are working together to create life from the bare savannah of silicon. Alife detractors are quick to point out that drawing evolutionary conclusions or vast conclusions from a small program would be an over simplification. Life in a bottle, even silicon, is not a realistic model (Van Winkle, W., 1998).

However, Tom Ray, a biologist at the University of Delaware and the ATR Human Information Processing Research Laboratories in Kyoto, Japan, has devised a solution. His brainchild, Tierra, spans hundreds of potentially millions of computers, all connected via the Internet. Each PC provides a small ecosystem for Tierra organisms, each of which contains only 32 instructions. But taken as a whole, the Internet provides the vast silicone landscape necessary for Ray's alife to evolve. Each organism is designed to replicate and compete for CPU and RAM space (the amount of space is predetermined by the Tierra software so as not to interfere with other system functions). When system resources become scarce, a "reaper" function kills off the old and malfunctioning organisms.

Mutations result from random flips in DNA code, which most often destroy the organism, but occasionally yield improvements. Tierra has developed parasites which shrink down to a single instruction unit and trick other organisms into expending their own CPU resources to copy it.

From speech recognition to architectural innovation, genetic programming promises to improve our world while accelerating ever more our rate of social and technological change (Epstein, J., Axtell, J., 1996).

3

A SAMPLE OF TOMORROW'S TECHNOLOGY

MIT's media lab is where some of the coolest new technologies are invented. (WWW.IBM Corporation Research). The lab is one of the few places where computers outnumber people by a significant margin. An experimental, gigabit fiber-optic plant connects a heterogeneous network of computers, ranging from fine-grained, embedded processors to super computers. The lab's growing rapid prototyping resources include 3-D printing, nano computing machine, injection of mold and PC board fabrication. There are also studies for audio, video, laboratory electromagnetic materials, optic and percepted studies. The Philippe Villors Experimental Media Facility, known as The Cube, provides a unique setting for large displays, acoustical studies and experimental performances (2000).

Overall, the lab consists of 28 departments, 227 graduate students, 154 under grads and 30 faculty members. Physically, the lab is divided up into several groups, each of which focuses on different types of inventions. The Tangible Media Group, for example, designs user interfaces which employ physical objects, surface and spaces as tangible embodiments of digital information. The overall goal is to converge the duel worlds of bits and atoms.

One thing the Tangible Media Group is currently focusing research on are smart rooms. Smart rooms would act like invisible butlers, using cameras, microphones, biosensors to interpret what people are doing and active agents to figure out how to help them. Potentially, smart rooms could be capable of recognizing who is in the room and interpreting their hand gestures.

A sampling of current research activities at MIT work under way at the Medial Laboratory with medical applications (WWW.IBM Corporation Research):

- Quantum computing—opens up the possibility that an ordinary liquid—like a cup of coffee—could harness natural forces so effectively that it would turn today's largest super computer into a digital dinosaur.

- Joining the physical environment and cyberspace—making "tangible bits" accessible through everyday physical surfaces like walls or desktops, and eventually through household surfaces like refrigerator doors.

- Full parallax holography—get the full effect of a hologram not only by looking side to side, but also by looking over and under the object. This work allows greater flexibility in design and permits the designer to place a model in a variety of environments.

Hospitals in the 21st century—Alternative medicine of today—smart rooms:

Stealth Platform for VR: The Surgical-Angio Suite, Workstations, Voice recognition, Hand recognition, Alife—DNA replica, percussor to cloning the human body, Bloodless knife, and teleportation.

FOREFRONT LEADERS

Stanford expects medical miracles with new "dream teams." Interdisciplinary research is one of the hottest trends in science. Stanford is assembling research "dream teams" to tackle the relationship between the "thinkers and the doers" (Konigsmark, A., 2000). How about a digital camera technology to "reprogram blind eyes to see" or how about a computer which is made of organic materials that's fed, not plugged-in. Or grow a new liver instead of transplanting one. The university has announced the first Bio-X research grants, signaling the start of studies using a combination of scientists, electrical engineers and computer scientists paired with doctors, physicists and biologists (Glausiusz, J., 1999).

Netscape co-founder Jim Clark gave Sanford $50 million to jump start. Bio-X, as it has been named, has set its goals. One of its first projects involves connecting a camera to retinal cells in a blind eye to develop a working nerve connection. This could lead to a cure age-related blindness. The establishment of interdisciplinary research with groups across the country could result in treatment and possibly cures for debilitating diseases. Trending the future of mankind, Bio-X and other research disciplines are open to new research grants in cross-departmental study proposals.

Bio-X is searching for new tools in analyzing the recent decoded human gene code; human tissue engineering (protein "chaperons," small proteins that help bigger ones fold and therefore function). Learning what goes on with smaller proteins could lead to cures for Alzheimer's, Huntington's and Parkinson's diseases. The connection between camera technology and the human eye could possibly lead to a pair of glasses equipped with a camera that photographs the world and delivers it to the retina. Relationships between B-cell lymphoma and vaccines that are designed for individual patients in as little time as a week. Stanford expects medical miracles and offers new interdisciplinary positions in Bio-X to focus on dreams of discovery in 2001.

DNA Sciences, Inc. are dealing with very powerful interventions in human destiny. Geron Corporation in Menlo Park, the company that developed a method for indefinitely extending the life of cells taken from human embryos. The Geron Company holds the rights to the cloning technology that created Dolly the Sheep. Key issues in bioethics today are the use of cells harvested from human embryos and fetuses; botched experiences to correct inherited defects with gene therapy and effects to identify individual genetic differences. Researchers predict the likelihood of future disease. DNA Sciences from Geron burst into public view with the announcement this summer that it would use the Internet to seek thousands of volunteers to donate their DNA to the for-profit company, which plans to use it to identify genes that play a role in more than 20 different diseases.

The firm's scientific and financial pedigree is impeccable. James D. Watson, co-discoverer of the structure of DNA, is on its board of directors, as well as Raymond L. White, a pioneer in mapping the human gene code. Among its financial backers is Jim Clark, founder of Silicon Graphics, Inc. and Netscape Communication Corp.

SAMPLE 1: ULTRACISION

The Ultracision scalpel seals as it makes incisions. Vibrating at 55,000 times per second, the blade generates ultrasound waves that change the nature of the proteins in tissue, so the tissue becomes sticky and coagulated to stop bleeding. The scalpel is currently being used at Cornell Medical Center in New York (Popular Science, 1998).

Company: Ethicon Endo-Surgery, 4545 Creek Road, Cincinnati, Ohio 45242.

SAMPLE 2: ONE WORLD, ONE LANGUAGE

Language continues to be a predominant barrier for people from other cultures and countries. The goal of Language Force, an Orange, California based software development company whose mission is to create "one world, one language." The company's first product was the Universal Translator Standard, introduced in 1997, which can translate 25 languages from Farsi to Thai—with the push of a button (Tokita, J. 1999).

The translation technology used in Language Force comes from the Soviet Space Agency. One of the co-founders of the company, Yuri Mordovoskoi, is a former major in the Russian military who holds a doctorate in artificial intelligence with an emphasis on linguistics. Mordovoskoi is the brains behind the company's technology.

Language Forces latest software, Instant Language 2000, Version 2.0. uses Speak and Hear technology. Now users can speak their own language and have it translated as they speak to someone else. Users can vocally interact with other languages via Internet. The software also comes with a translation pad that allows user to type in English words and phrases, instantly translates them into another language—restricted to Spanish, French, German or Russian at this time. With its point and speak feature, you can point to any word or phrase you see on any website and hear the pronunciation in English or any one of the other languages available (Tokita, J., 1999)

SAMPLE 3: THE NEXT GENERATION NEURONAVIGATION SYSTEM

Currently, the U.S. Air Force has technology available for fighter pilots that projects information into their field-of-view so they do not have to shift their eyes to see it. In an effort to bring this technology into their surgery suite, Wallace-Kettering, Neuroscience Institute in Dayton, Ohio, has formed a joint project with nearby Wright Patterson Air Force Base. Microvision, Inc. of Seattle has signed on with the project. It will incorporate virtual retinal display (VRD) into a computer-guided neurosurgical navigation system that will enable the surgeon to use images and visual cues during surgery without having to look up from the field or microscope. One goal of the research collaboration is to perfect a small, unobtrusive projector that will sit on the physician's glasses and display images directly on their retina (Ward, J., 1998).

The project, called "The Next Generation Neuronavigation System," is under the direction of Martin Sattler, Ph.D., a positron emission tomography (PET) physicist at Wallace Kettering. "The project entails inputs from many devices (microscopes, C-arms, etc.) typically utilized in a brain or spine surgery into the neuronavigation computer system for output to the VRD. This will allow a wide range of information (physiologic, images, video) to be transmitted to the neuro-surgeon in a non-perturbing manner through the VRD system."

Gerald Szkotruck, MHA, executive director of Wallace-Kettering Neuro-science Institute, believes the many breakthroughs in various techniques lead to reliance on image guidance during surgery. At this time, progress has been made to update imaging by having the computed tomography (CT) or MRI in the surgery suite actually taking the images (Ward, J., 1998).

"Another way to work in computer techniques using certain markers defined in the PET, CT or MRI scan. These images could be updated digitally to allow for the surgical changes. These images also can be combined with the updated CT or MRI offering a combination of techniques. There is also an interest in using a hand held positron marker, which would indicate the presence of tumor cells.

The ideas is to have this technology in image-guided assistant for the neuro-surgeon to use anytime by just pushing on a foot pedal or using a voice command. The surgeon can then bring up PET image and have it scanned and overlaid right in the image of the patient's anatomy so that it can be referenced without having to lift their eyes from the field or the microscope.

Another area under exploration is the use of the infrared camera during surgery. Tumor tissue has a slightly higher metabolism than normal tissue that may be detectable with a specialized infrared camera.

This current project was initiated several years ago when a number of public officials were invited to tour Wallace-Kettering. "We were demonstrating co-registration of medical images; this generated a great deal of interest in developing the technology further," Szkototnicki said. "The officials at Wright-Patterson Air Force Base expressed interest in assisting us with technology transfer. Basically, the idea was to create a new technology combining some of the resources available locally. Eventually a package was put together between us and the Department of Defense."

Researchers at Wallace-Kettering decided to invite Microvision into the research partnership because the company had already made significant progress on a display technique that uses laser retinal scanning. Szkotnicki said, "An important part of the project is to make the image display as light and unobtrusive as possible. In this device, VGA-type is scanned using a small blue laser directly on the user's retina. It is something that is very light and small" (Ward, J., 1998).

SAMPLE 4: IMAGING THE NEW MILLENNIUM

Much of today's imaging technology still relies on invasive techniques—the use of ionization radiation, injected or ingested contrast media and radioisotopes, incision or orifice insertion of scopes, and directed sonics and radio frequency energies. Medical imaging of the future will be largely non-invasive (Strauss, J. & Horli, S., 1995).

Advances in medical imaging already have reduced the need for most highly invasive exploratory surgeries. Patient safety has been improved by the approximate 50% reduction in radiation exposure afforded by rare earth screens and faster films. Subsequently, development of digital detectors, such as storage phosphor imaging plates, provided further opportunities for dose reduction.

The most significant development in imagery combined with treatment in the growth of minimally invasive surgical techniques made possible by devices that provide internal imaging and obviate the need for large incisions to visualize the anatomy. Examples are found in the management of gallstones, as laparoscopic cholecystectomy has virtually replaced open cholecystectomy for cholelithiasis. Cholelithiasis is increasingly treated with therapeutic biliary endoscopy over surgical common bile duct exploration.

Medical imaging in the next century will explore entirely new pathways. New "signaling" or imaging generated sources will be required to provide a broader range of information than the anatomical information currently provided to satisfy the need for a more efficient and definitive diagnostic process, "quantum mirage" (Piller, C., 2000).

Extension of current functional imaging will occur by using novel imaging agents produced through genetic engineering methods. Molecular tags that alter magnetic resonance, ultrasound, or intrinsic signals could be attached to substrates to follow metabolic activity or alter it. This is not far from radio-nuclide imaging, but the molecular probes could be designed using genetic engineering techniques to target specific cells, genetic material, or metabolic processes and do so without radioactive isotopes.

New detectors will be developed that are naturally occurring signal-sources emanating from the body as the input. Sophisticated detectors will passively use the electrical, thermal, chemical, acoustic, and visual emissions of the body to create anatomic as well as physiologic and pathologic data sets for improved diagnosis. The technology and science of sensing the body as a dynamic signal source may come to be known as "physiological signal imaging," wearable computers placed on the body for tracting (Page, D., 2000).

Developments in "nano-technology" could have a major impact on medical imaging. Image acquisition, a bit more invasive than looking at passive signals, would employ micro-machines that could be displayed in the bloodstream or directly injected into the area of interest. These could provide direct (through nanosensors) and indirect imaging of microscopic anatomy. By sensing and responding to local biochemical variation, they could also provide images of in vivo "smart" micro machines that coordinate action via an external, macro computing system, both diagnostic and therapeutic procedures could be performed (Hatfield, S., 1998).

Nano-technology also could be used for support of displays, the limitations of cathode ray tubes (CRTs) are well known. Nano-technology fabricated flat panel displays (micro-mirror systems and field-emission panels are but two examples), could easily surpass CRTs in both spatial and contrast resolutions. Of course, direct viewing of visual displays may itself be superseded. Virtual reality systems couple visual displays much closer to the eye. Closer yet would display systems directly coupled to the visual cortex of the brain, either semi-invasively with microelectrode systems, or non-invasively through conditioned signals applied to the scalp. This would bypass both the eye and its associated neural nuclei, but could function in conjunction with conventional vision to permit guided procedures with stimulated cortical imagery "super imposed" on the visual field (Hatfield, S., 1997).

World wide databases analysis will accelerate the development of a knowledge pool essential for the advance of the associated diagnostic science. In addition, artificial intelligence systems will be in wide use in many decision systems. They will likely provide the initial, primary diagnosis in medical imaging.

Detecting the body's own emanations and those of smart machines will provide a nearly non-invasive approach to imaging. This will provide a more civilized approach to imaging in the future that would simplify the examination process through reduced costs, lower risk and increased access. The availability of low cost but sophisticated signaling technology and analysis will enable the creation of home "wellness pods" and walk-in diagnostic kiosks (Strauss, J. & Horli, S., 1995).

SAMPLE 5: BLOODLESS SURGERY

Gamma Knife technology allows surgery without a scalpel or incision. With extreme precision, Sutter Gamma Knife Radiosurgery Center physicians are able to operate on the brain or skull with minimal risk of surgical complications and with less damage to surrounding tissue. Sutter Health is one of the few hospital systems providing this procedure that has revolutionized brain surgery (Griffith, D., 1998).

The Gamma Knife is not a knife at all. Rather, it is a technologically advanced, 20-ton machine that allows surgeons to delivery 201 beams of ionizing gamma rays, precisely targeting the treatment area. Replacing the need for the combination of conventional brain surgery and intensive radiation treatment. Gamma Knife technology delivers enough radiation to destroy tumors or arteriovenous malformations while minimizing damage to surrounding normal tissue.

In 1949, Lars Leksell, M.D., Ph.D. (1907-1986), introduced his stereotactic instrument to the medical world. The original Gamma Knife radiosurgery tool, the Leksell Microstereotactic System, instantly occupied a unique position as the world's leading instrument for stereotactic neurosurgery.

The Gamma Knife is especially valuable for patients whose neurologic disorders require a different surgical approach or may be impossible by conventional neurosurgical techniques. Patients of advanced age or in poor medical condition can be at an unacceptable high risk for anesthesia and conventional surgery.

Dr. Michael S. Edwards, Medical Director of the new Sutter Gamma Knife Radiosurgery Center, states "the development of sophisticated imaging studies and sophisticated computer planning programs now make this machine far more accurate, reliable, and useful for neurosurgery."

Magnetic resonance imaging, PET scans or angiograms are used to pinpoint the targeted tumor or lesion. Using this information and patient medical history, patients who otherwise may not get through a major operation because of a bad heart, can undergo surgery and have a good prognosis.

It also is used for treating vascular malformations in areas of the brain where traditional surgery could cause brain damage, and to treat disorders such as Parkinson's disease by destroying areas within the brain that are responsible for abnormal movements of the extremities.

Clinical Studies:

A noninvasive radiosurgical-technique may ultimately replace surgery for many patients with Parkinson's disease and other movement disorders whose symptoms cannot be controlled by medicine, according to the results of a preliminary study presented during the annual meeting of the Radiological Society of North America (RSNA). Stereotactic radiosurgery is performed with equipment called a gamma knife that uses magnetic resonance (MR) imaging to identify the radiosurgical target. The radiation destroys selected portions of the globus pallidus on the thalamus, structures deep within the brain that are responsible for the tumors and other involuntary movements that are characteristic of Parkinsons disease.

Sutter expects to treat 80 to 100 patients the first year, beginning in October, 1999, after testing the apparatus and training additional neurosurgeons and radiation oncologists to use it. Each procedure will cost between $20,000 and $30,000 (Griffith, D., 1998).

Dr. David Larson, co-director of the gamma knife facility at UCSF—Stanford Health Care, said he is not concerned that another gamma knife is in Northern California. The Sutter program also should not interfere with the U.C. Davis Medical Center's stereotactic linear accelerator radiosurgery, said Dr. John Earle, radiation oncology chair . That technology is best used for tumors that are diffuse and infiltrating. The gamma knife is the best choice for tumors that are small, deep and close to the vital parts of the brain.

Radiosurgery provides effective treatment of intra cranial lesions such as: Acoustic neuromas, arteriovenous malformations, brain stem tumors, chordomas, craniopharyngiomas, meningiomas, metastases, movement disorders, pineal tumors, pituitary adenomas, primary glial tumors, and trigeminal neuralgia.

SAMPLE 6: TECHNOLOGY OF THE YEAR

Industry Week recently named the amorphous silicon technology used in GE Medical Systems' new digital x-ray detector, one of its "25 Technologies of the Year." Designed and developed at GE's Research and Development Center in Schenectady, New York, the Digital X-ray Detector technology was designed to replace conventional x-ray film and chemicals with computer images that can be electronically or sent anywhere in the world via telecommunications technology.

This technology is currently under clinical investigation and is the basis of an entirely new category of G.E. medical products that produce x-ray images of the breast, chest, heart, blood vessels, bone, and abdomen without film (Kasler, D., 1998).

Toshiba America Medical Systems (TAMS) announced that Charles Corogenes has been named director, CT Business Unit. Corogenes is responsible for the designing and implementing of strategic marketing programs to support Toshiba's product offerings. These products include the industry's first real-time CT scanning technology. Aspire continuous imaging (CI), which eliminates blend exams and can reduce procedure time by 50 to 90%; Sure Start, a contrast monitoring system which can reduce contract use by 25%; and C.T. port, a CT radiation therapy simulation product which streamlines cancer therapy.

"With more than 24 years of experience in the radiology industry, Mr. Corogenes has been a valuable asset to the CT Business Unit and Toshiba," said John Zimmer, Vice President, Marketing. "True to his extensive background in sales, service, and radiology department management, we believe Mr. Corogenes will continue to provide CT technologies which meet the U.S. health care market's needs by emphasizing improvements in patient care, efficiency, and cost containment" (Kasler, D., 1998).

SAMPLE 7: TOMORROW'S INFORMATION STRUCTURE

Defining Tomorrow's Information Structure

The 611 Awards recognize those who are using the Internet and networking technology to produce extraordinary results (Poulos, C., 1998).

The Global Information Infrastructure (GII) Awards are different—"a cross between the Oscars and the Baldridge Awards of the Internet" by USA Today, the GII Awards recognize champions across all industries and sectors of society who are using the Internet and network technology to produce extraordinary results—the people and organizations who are defining tomorrow's information infrastructure today.

The GII Awards, a non-partisan and independent initiative, has been cited by Vice President Gore as "an innovation that is vital to our country's future." In eleven categories GII Awards will go to individuals, businesses and organizations who are using the information superhighways in collaborative innovation and results oriented ways.

What makes a project innovative? It is the dedication to finding new ways to use technology to serve, educate, entertain or provide services to the users.

As an example, the University of California, San Diego's Collaboratory for Microscopy and Digital Anatomy (<http://www-nemir-ucsd.edu/CMDAA/7), this project allows scientists and researchers from around the world access to a one-of-a-kind microscope and powerful computers that otherwise would only have been available to a select few.

Another project of innovated magnus is Deployable Radiology to support U.S. troops in Bosnia (iterzegovina<http://www.1mac.georgetown.edu/bosma/start.html7), state-of-the-art mobile diagnostic equipment.

According to William Van Winkle, author of "Artificial Life: Will Technology Create Artificial Life?" (1998), after many millennia of struggle, we humans pride ourselves on being on top of the food chain, God's chosen species. We are complex in a way that no animal could emulate—so complex, in fact, that we pay therapists thousands of dollars a year to sort out our crossed wires.

A common Creationist argument runs that evolution cannot exist because no one ever sees it happening. (Has anyone ever seen an ape change into a human?) This is a very limited view—but points to understanding evolutionary processes, both in the past and the extrapolating into the future.

The minuscule gene changes which fuel a species-wide metamorphosis take tens of thousands, sometimes millions of years to become noticeable. If only there were a process to accelerate these changes.

Enter artificial life, or "alife." Working from the model that gene code is analogous to computer code, several groups are working to create life from the base savannah of silicon. One of the first and most recognized was the "Sugarscape" program developed by Joshua M. Epstein and Robert Axtell at the Brookings Institution in Washington, D.C.

Sugarscape Secrets: As Science New reported (November 23, 1996), Sugarscape is a virtual world, a two-dimensional grid inhabited by basic software "agents" and certain resources which the agents need to survive.

In the simplest, there are two areas high in "sugar" resource, which can grow back after being consumed. Agents search as far as vision permits, find the unoccupied spot with the most sugar, go there, and eat the sugar." Basic hunter-gatherer philosopher.

Interestingly, recognizable trends begin to form when population rises. A minority of agents with better vision and lower mechanisms accumulate most of the sugar. The less fortunate majority often subsists in the sugar scrubland. Some die of starvation.

Alife detractors are quick to point out that drawing evolutionary conclusion from a small program is over simplification. Thus, life in a bottle, they say, even a silicone one, simply is not a realistic model.

However, Tom Ray, a biologist at the University of Delaware and the ATR Human Information Processing Research Laboratories in Kyoto, Japan, has devised a solution. His brainchild, Tierra, spans hundreds and potentially millions of computers; all connected via the Internet. Each PC provides a small ecosystem for Tierra organisms, each of which only contains 32 instructions. But taken as a whole, the Internet provides the vast silicon landscape necessary for Ray's alife to evolve. Each organism is designed to replicate and compete for CPU and Ramscope. The amount of space is predetermined as not to interfere with other system functions. When the system resources become scarce, a "reaper" function kills off the old and malfunctioning organisms.

Mutations result from random flips in DNA code, which most often destroy the organism, but occasionally yield improvements. Tierra has developed parasites which shrink down to a single instruct or unit and trick other organisms into expending their own CPU resources to copy it. Predators have suddenly emerged. More interestingly, a primitive form of sex, in which organisms swap code to reproduce, has evolved. This may, in time, shed light on the unanswered questions of why sex, not necessarily present in lower life forms, exists in the first place. Ray hopes to make Tierra environment available to anyone with Internet access.

Ultimately, the potential discoveries which alife may yield are well worth the possibility of encountering yet another "virus." The Cyrix-based Pentium, straining under 32 MB of RAM may provide a much more hostile environment (Macintosh or Pentium II). Alife is one manifestation of a field you are going to hear more about. From speech recognition to architectural innovation, genetic programming promises to improve our world while accelerating ever more our rate of social and technological change.

William Van Winkle is a freelance writer who specializes in futuristic technologies, believes as a collective, human life continues to undergo stress and mutations, perhaps the most appropriate instructor we can find to help us understand these transformations are our digital brethren (Van Winkle, 1998).

SAMPLE 8: DNA CHIPS

Affymetrix, Inc., a promising young biotechnology company from Santa Clara is readying a $10 million dollar plant that will manufacture an ingenious hybrid of semi conductors and genetics called GeneChip (Kasler, D., 1999). A glass wafer coated with DNA, the GeneChip could enable Affymetrix's customers—some of the world's leading pharmaceutical companies—to develop breakthrough treatments for cancer, AIDS and other diseases.

The West Sacramento plant, scheduled to open in late summer or early fall, will give the company the ability to make chips in large volumes, a crucial development that show Affymetrix has matured well. It could represent an important transition for the Sacramento area.

Area officials hope Affymetrix can help spark the region's fledgling biotechnology industry joining such companies as Mansanto, industrial-enzyme firm Novo Nordisk Biotech, Inc., pesticide maker AgraQuest Inc. and Seminis Vegetalie Seeds in Woodland with the University of California, Davis. Affymetrix shows signs that it wants to use its vast research base as a tool for regional economic development, many officials believe the Sacramento area could be on the verge of a biotech explosion.

Research and development functions will remain in Santa Clara, the West Sacramento plant will focus strictly on chip manufacturing.

The sample seeps onto the DNA subsiding on the chip. Then chemistry will take over. The DNA from the sample will end with the DNA on the chip in a certain precise fashion.

The chip is then scanned by a Hewlett-Packard Co. measuring device, providing a readout that enables the researcher to analyze gene mutations that might have led to the disease. DNA from a cancerous tissue, for instance, will mate with the GeneChip in such a way that "you could identify these specific genes that might be involved in the particular cancer."

GeneChip analysis could help pharmaceutical companies design new drugs or enable GeneChip to see wether a particular drug is still effective on a particular gene. Analyzing genes is nothing new, but until recently scientists could analyze only a handful of genes at a time. The Affymetrix system can analyze thousands of genes at a clip.

Even so, Affymetrix customers have to buy the chips in mass quantities. The West Sacramento plant will have the capacity to manufacture 1 million to 3 million chips a year. The cheapest Affymetrix chips sells for about $90; the most expensive can cost thousands. That is peanuts compared to the whole GeneChip system, including the measuring instrumentation and the equipment that mates the GeneChip with the tissue samples. The entire system is just under $200,000.

The price has not been too rich for Affymetrix's big-time customers. They include Warner-Lambert's Parke-Davis Pharmaceutical Division, Hoechst Marion Roussel Inc. And F. Hoffman-La Roche Ltd. (Kasler, D., 1999).

British pharmaceutical firm Glaxo Willcome Plc. has gone one step further, amassing a 36.9 percent stake in Affymetrix according to records filed with the Securities and Exchange Commission. The Affymetrix stock price has more than doubled since September; its market valuation totals $814 million. Not too bad for a company that has yet to turn a profit. In 1998, it lost $23.1 million on sales of $52 million; in 1997, the company dropped $22.5 million on sales of $19.8 million. The losses are not at all discouraging for a biotech company that is barely six years old. They expect to become profitable next year.

SAMPLE 9: AGING AMERICA

It appears that the Republican Congress will abide by its contract with America and propose cuts to reduce the federal deficit. However, there is an alternative which may delay the controversial slashing of Medicare funds: Medicare HMOs. Medicare HMOs are Congress' way of relieving a top-heavy federal program by transferring arrangement is that for each beneficiary enrolled, HCFA reimburses the HMO at the rate of 95% of the amount paid for the average Medicare beneficiary. The rate is based on a five-year average and is paid monthly. In return, the HMO agrees to provide all the medical care for the enrollees. The HMO is permitted to charge its members a premium, although in saturated markets the level of competition may prevent it from doing so. Because Medicare HMOs receive only 95% of Medicare allowances, out of which they must also pay their administrative costs, they are unable to reimburse participating physicians at 100% of the general Medicare rate (Boland, P., 1993). Benefits of Medicare HMO:

1. The federal government is relieved of having to manage the continually rising costs of health care for the elderly and at a 5% discount at that.

2. Medicare HMOs develop only in communities with surplus of physicians. Therefore, in return for a lower reimbursement rate, physicians are guaranteed a steady flow of patients.

3. Patients like the fact that they are no longer responsible for a 20% co-pay.

Medicare HMOs have their imperfections for physicians but if they join one they can increase the size of their practice while reducing the size of the federal deficit (Boland, P., 1993).

SAMPLE 10: SOCIO ECONOMICS OF IMAGING.

Trinity Hospital, a 40-bed rural hospital in Erin, Tennessee, was facing a number of challenges in providing specialized medical care to the community. Trinity Hospital, like many small rural hospitals, did not have the best reputation for service and was losing too many patients to Clarksville, forty miles away (Elliot, J., 1989).

Jack Buck, chief executive officer at Trinity Hospital, became intrigued with the possibilities that telemedicine could provide. He heard that rural hospitals could not afford telemedicine. Buck decided to attend a presentation made by a medical systems integration organization, Telemed, on the role telemedicine would play in rural health care.

A system integrator's expertise is in "linking" large hospitals via telecommunications lines to regional and rural hospitals. They typically offer a comprehensive range of telemedicine systems, integration strategic planning, needs assessment, applications, services design, specifically for the unique diagnostic and information needs of health care organizations.

Convinced that telemedicine would benefit Trinity, Buck developed several goals that he wanted to accomplish with such a system. He needed to attract more physicians to the hospital, convince patients to stay locally rather than drive 40 miles to Clarksville or 120 miles to Nashville, improve his census count and technical fees while keeping costs low.

The implementation of telemedicine was made possible through private funding from the rural hospital budget, and a radiology group, RCI. The 18-member radiology group in Nashville had never dealt with teleradiology, but had provided outstanding service to physicians at their large flagship hospital, Columbia/Centennial, and possessed a wealth of subspecialty expertise.

The system integrator was able to connect Trinity Hospital and RCI to a high speed, secure ATM network backbone. RCI had already chosen a vendor for their teleradiology equipment, but needed someone to help with integrating it into their workflow system. More importantly, they needed someone to come up with solutions to provide remote dictation and remote fluoroscopy. The integrator also assisted with the implementation of RCI's diagnostic quality imaging, so the radiologists could provide a primary diagnosis within minutes over the telecommunications link.

"Before we adopted our teleradiology program, we had to transport radiology exams 70 miles by courier before a radiologist could review them and provide a diagnosis," Brick explained, "With teleradiology we have the diagnosis almost instantaneously and can proceed with treatment more rapidly." (Elliot, J., 1989.)

Trinity had been receiving radiology services two hours a day, two days a week, as part of the network. Interactive video technology allows the radiology group to perform remote fluoroscopy and CT scans sevens days a week, rather than only when the radiologist is on site.

"The change in service levels for rural physicians was immediate and noticeable. They were amazed by the support they were now getting. It was service-oriented and really worked to build the radiologists' relationships with the rural physicians." Buck said.

With telemedicine, Buck was able to attract six additional staff physicians including an orthopedist, podiatrist, pediatrics ob/gyn, and a general surgeon, and three family practitioners. Physicians who were being squeezed out of the larger markets by competition and managed care were able to move to a rural setting, have a better family life and endure less competition (Elliot, J., 1989).

As predicted, Trinity Hospital has grown at a staggering rate. Trinity's market share has risen from 24% to 74% in two years. The hospital's outpatient census has grown 25 percent, with additional growth in its patient base. Outpatient visits at Trinity have grown from 600 per month to more than 1,100 per month in one year, and its bottom line revenues have increased by $250,000, far exceeding the cost of the system.

Trinity is now considering a top-notch facility in the area, and was recently recognized as among the top 10 percent of Columbia facilities in quality patient care. They have been so successful that they are now opening clinics in Clarksville to draw patients to Trinity, and plan to expand the telemedicine system to include cardiology in the near future.

With collaboration, maneuvering around obstacles, Trinity Hospital has proven cost effective and provides excellent patient care. When presented with similar challenges, rural hospitals that implement the proper technological solution can make a positive change which the entire community can appreciate.

4

CONCLUSION

With managed care in the driver seat, look for U.S. digital x-ray market to double over the next six years. That's the projection from market research firm Frost & Sullivan (Mountain View, California) in its latest report, which estimates that the U.S. digital market will reach $1.5 million by 2004, based on an anticipated compound annual growth rate of 8 percent.

"Managed care is motivating providers to decrease costs and increase efficiency," said Ryan Goulding, medical imaging consultant at Frost & Sullivan and author of the report. Managed care has also made it clear that providers are in competition with one another, so factors that can distinguish one provider from another provider are a facility's respective assets. Digital x-ray becomes a tremendous tool, the report stated, to bolster marketing effects and increase the quality and breadth of services (Ayers, J. & Benson, L., 1995).

SHORT-STAY SURGERY

During the recent years, short-stay surgery or day surgery has become increasingly normal. In the United States, more than 47% of all surgical procedures are performed in ambulatory surgery programmes, in which people do not remain in the hospital overnight after surgery compared to only 20% in 1983. By the year 2000 as much as two-thirds of all surgery could be done in ambulatory settings (Davis, J. E., 1987).

Most procedures making up Minimal Invasive Technology (MIT) are still performed with hospitalization, at least in Europe. However, in the United States in part because of financial pressures to reduce hospitalization rate, MIT may be carried out more often as a day surgery treatment. For example, many groups in the United States are performing laparoscopic cholecystectomy with good results without hospital admission. In Europe, MIT is generally not seen as a way to reduce the need for hospital beds. Day surgery seems both economically advantageous to patients and to society (Banter, 1992).

The most important implication of MIT is for patients. In the Netherlands, it has been demonstrated that laser palliation of colon cancer is associated with less use of hospital beds than conventional surgery (Matthews, R., 1994).

As has already been emphasized, these procedures cause less trauma to the patient. They are generally associated with less morbidity, less pain, and an earlier return to normal activities. It seems apparent that patients should have a choice of these new therapies when they have been shown to be effective. However, physicians often decide for patients. Patients can only ask for these new procedures if they know that they exist.

MIT has important implications for physicians. In some cases, specialities are changing. Interventional radiology has developed as radiologists have seen the possibilities of treatment in conjunction with imaging methods.

General surgery has gradually lost much of its work through technological changes and shifts to other specialities. This particular speciality may essentially disappear or merge with internal medicine. The endoscopist, who is often presently an internist, can look directly into the body at many lesions—with increased treatment practices on the spot, by wire loop, laser vaporization, heater probe, and other technology. New treatment, provided proper research has been conducted, will seek the gene chip.

The Stealth Platform is capable of adding up to seven, possibly up to eleven, major digital equipment tools. The MIT system will change the future of surgical procedures—smart rooms such as surgical-angio suites, endoscopic diagnosis, micro-endoscopic treatments, 3-D imaging, integration of medical information systems, mini-clusters of technological scanning—mobile C arm, MRI, CRT, US, duplex scans, nuclear medicine, PET, lasers—with an infinite number of applications (Hatfield, S., 1998).

The Sugarscape project—research for Alternative Medical Practices as an answer to diagnosis, treatment and possible a cure for diseases.

Cloning, pharming, artificial intelligence, CAD, retina scanning, voice recognition, hand sensors, bloodless knife, 3-D patient plan, and DNA research all available for tomorrow's hospitals. Within a decade, scientists aim to create transplantable human hearts (Stover, D., 1994). Doctors have joined forces with engineers and biochemists to assemble living cells into spare parts for the human body. A consortium of tissue engineers is attempting to grow a heart in a box. Biodegradable scaffolding on which to grow human tissue has been around since the mid-1980's, but researchers are experimenting with the shapes and materials that can be used to optimize cell growth (Sukthankar, M., 1994).

Seeded with starter cells, a scaffolding is suspended around a bio reactor that supplies the cells with oxygen and nutrients. During the last few years scientists have created individual components of the heart such as arteries, valves, and muscle tissue. Perhaps the most far-reaching project is an initiative called Living Implants From Engineering (LIFE), led by Michael Sefton, director of the Institute of Biomaterials and Biomedical Engineering of the University of Toronto (1998).

The LIFE consortium includes researchers from MIT, Massachusetts General Hospital, the Pittsburgh Tissue Engineering Initiative, and other facilities in the United States, Canada, Europe, and Japan, plan on building a heart within a decade. Sefton estimates that creating a fully functional heart for pre-clinical testing with cost $5 billion. It is though that "If we can figure out how to engineer a heart, the rest of the organs will follow," says Sefton (Sefton, 1998).

First, researchers create a scaffolding with the three-dimensional shape of the tissue they are engineering. Scaffoldings are typically made from biodegradable polymers such as polylactic acid and polyglycolic acid, originally developed for sutures. The next step is to seed the scaffolding with the cells taken from the type of organ the researchers hope to create. The cell studded scaffolding is placed in a bioreactor which is kept at body temperature, a mixture of oxygenated nutrients is pumped around and through the scaffolding. The cells divide and secrete proteins and growth factors that bind them together to form living tissue. Dr. Joseph Vacanti, a professor of surgery at Harvard Medical School and Massachusetts General Hospital, and Robert Langer, a chemical engineering professor at MIT, are among the fathers of tissue engineering.

Vacanti has used this method to create 27 different types of tissue in his lab alone. The first useful products were small sheets of skin and pieces of cartilage fashioned into recognizable shapes such as noses and ears.

Other researchers have created whole organs. At Harvard Medical School, Dr. Anthony Atala has grown bladders from dogs using their own cells. Tissue engineers are setting their sights on complex organs. They already create rudimentary blood vessels, valves and muscles. Some teams have created "artificial arteries" by growing smooth muscle cells on a polymer tube and then coating the inside of the tube with epithelial lining cells. Clogging is an even more serious problem for smaller blood vessels. To create the blood supply for a heart, researches will have to design tiny, branding capillaries. The biotechnology company Organogenesis in Canton, Massachusetts is working on a possible solution: creating blood vessels from natural collagen (the body's connective tissue) coated with a layer of antico-agulant that prevents clogs. Once implanted, the tubes attract the body's own vascular cells and grow into normal blood vessels. David Mooney, an associate professor of biologic and materials science at the University of Michigan, is seed-ing cells onto scaffoldings clamped to mechanical devices that repeatedly tug on the scaffoldings as the tissue develops (Sefton, 1998).

Dr. Joseph Vacanti is also looking at a new way of fabricating scaffoldings. His idea is to use micro fabrication techniques borrowed from the computer industry to make a "tissue on a chip," with structures that are fractions of a micron in size, but made from biomaterial instead of silicon. Preserving the heart is a major problem. Freezing is the most likely method to keep the tissue alive until trans-plant. When cells thaw cracking occurs. Unless the heart in a box can be made from the patients own cells, recipients will have the same problems of immune rejection they encounter with today's transplant.

To grow the components of a human heart in a lab, some researchers are turn-ing to high-tech equipment. The bioreactor used to incubate engineered tissue are derived from the rotating wall bioreactor developed by NASA for micro grav-ity experiments. The rotating ensures even distribution of the nutrients through-out the scaffolding.

Creating the biodegradable scaffolding that support growing cells is a job made for another tool, a three-dimensional printer, 3DP. Patented in 1993 by a group at MIT led by mechanical engineer Emanuel Sachs, the 3DP was originally developed to create instant prototypes of parts for airplanes and other machines, e.g. ceramic molds for metal castings.

Biomedical engineer Linda Griffith of MIT is using 3DP to make body parts. First, she creates a computerized blueprint for the scaffolding and sends it to the 3DP. The printer's multiple link-jet nozzles then spit out micro drops of a glue-like binder onto an ultrathin layer of a powdered biodegradable polymer. The micro drops bind with the powder and solidify. The process is repeated, layer upon layer, until the sequence directed by the blueprint completes the entire structure. Engineering tissue such as a heart valve can be grown on biodegradable scaffoldings created by a 3-D printer.

An engineering coronary artery could eliminate the need to remove a major vessel from a patient's leg for bypass surgery. A piece of engineered chunk of heart tissue could be useful for testing drugs. Already one potential spin-off is a cardiac "patch" that could replace tissue damaged by a heart attack.

Ultimately, stem cells—the precursor cells that differentiate to form various organs—may make the job easier, if scientists could figure out the biochemical trigger that cause stem cells to turn into heart cells. Other bio tech labs have grown bladders for dogs (www.popsci.com) and "artificial" skin for sale (www.popsci.com).

A PLACE IN THE MODERN WORLD

Technically speaking, analysis might be better to classify decision-making as an intuitive art or science that can correlate elements, data, goals, visions, and meaningful conclusions that require patience for detail, open mindedness and the capacity to reason. Modern science and partly intuitive discipline will not over emphasize predictions, but might describe the general effect of current or future cycles, trends and interpretation of better education. The ability to use tools and concepts from related fields provides a method of analysis which helps promote growth.

Artificial Intelligent displays are adherent to weakness and limitation. Attempts to predict the future are too broad and leave a lasting pattern of disbelief. Artificial Intelligent display projects information without becoming unduly entangled in the state of doubt and apprehension. New tools for discovery are marvels of the age of science and electronics.

We should make use of the knowledge and symbols at hand, just as the Greeks, Chinese, and other ancients were able to perceive truths using the tools and concepts of their own time. True scientists perceive the limits of their own knowledge, and they know that their knowledge is eternally limited by time. The researchers need all the wisdom of the past, from every land, to augment the future.

Circles, cycles, ages, are parables of time caused by sequences of signs in technology. Due to a larger number of people in the world science needs to create and solve complex problems at a global level. We are never outside the path of inherent predictable patterns of change. The weaker standards of the past must yield to the right of way to the future. That is why the present is difficult for man.

A new age of technologies spin rapidly, moving away from old medical practices towards new ones. These technologies have more to do with revolution and less with evolution. The lack of current accurate investigation, lack of information to loss of perspective contribute to research for change on a larger scale in medicine.

Intuitive speculative thinking is a supercognitive process which allows an individual to synthesize, observe, all perceptions, then amplify the power of continuous research in new ways to develop better medical technology to be used in the coming Millennium.

BALANCING HEMICYCLES

The Information Age is moving forward into the high-technical age based on quarter time circle for review, revise, re-engineer, expansion, reallocation of resources and balancing financial contracts.

Major research programs set by Stanford, University of San Diego Medical School, Harvard, and Mayo Clinic, had notable findings. Each study represents a compelling reason to develop a graduate school to associate curriculum with contracts and synchronize new radiology technology [Telemedicine, speech recognitiion, global society, spiral C.T. and virtual reality (Hatfield, S., 1997), C.T. and Fluroscopy (Ward, J., 1999), Cardiovascular with C.T. and MRI (Hatfield, S., 1999), PACS (Kyes, K., 1995)]

5

SUMMARY

For the broad society MIT's research is so valuable, resources can be saved and allocated for future health care. So far, policy makers, insurers, and hospitals have been slow to recognize this potential. Hospitals and insurance companies tend to define cost effectiveness, efficiency and profit from their own perspective. Researchers recognize technological change.

1. Funding to stimulate development in technology which proves to be cost-effective.

2. Payment methods that are more sensitive to hospitals and physicians for effectiveness, efficiency and better outcomes.

3. Certifications of institutions and individuals for carrying out new technological procedures.

4. Support training programs.

5. Government support research for new medical procedures.

6. Concerted efforts to improve access to research for health practices, so people have a better basis for choice.

The use of computers as diagnostic tools has had variable success in clinical practice. Artificial intelligence based systems for collection of patient histories and evaluation of differential diagnosis have been able to in some cases compete with experienced clinicians in terms of diagnostic accuracy. Artificial intelligence based interpretations of electrocardiograms on the other hand has become standard option of all modern electrocardiographic recorders. Most physicians do not use the interpretive results and recent studies have questioned the validity and accuracy of the interpretative programs.

An alternative approach to medical diagnostic has been the recent interest in using neural networks to solve clinical problems. Many of the previously difficult tasks, such as image interpretation and analysis of multiple streams of data in real time, have been successfully preformed using neural networks. These technologies are surprisingly accurate, and may prove beneficial to the analysis of complex clinical problems. (Smith, K. R., 1994).

The nature and objectives of any enterprise must be defined in a way that allows it to capitalize on new opportunities or consciously pass them by. The functions of a business must be re-examined in terms of the widest possible current and future markets. Innovation means more than the development and application of new concepts. It calls for the collateral and even precursive discarding of old concepts. Thus John Diebold (Heyel, C., 1972) has always been highly articulate about the overriding need for "rethinking" traditional ways of doing things if a business is to take full advantage of advancing technology.

John Diebold repeatedly pointed out to client groups and other professional audiences application of advanced technology production or data processing aspects of the business. He insisted that this is a problem for technologists—not for management (Heyel, C., 1972).

Rethinking must be done on an extremely broad basis—viewing the objectives of the entire organization as a whole. It cannot be confined to the product design or engineering department. It must be an attitude, a state of mind, permeating the entire organization. (Automation: The Advent of the Automatic Factory," Princeton, New Jersey, Van Nostrand Company, Inc., 1952)

A strategic assessment of the problems and opportunities inherent in social changes resulting from new technology in health care.

DEFINING THE REAL FUNCTION OF THE BUSINESS

Such esoteric concepts as "defining the real function of the business" may, John Diebold concedes, be intuitively understood by successful entrepreneurs. However, he adds, the high rate of product failure indicates that they may be more widely misunderstood. The essence of the approach called for, as he sees it, is (1) a sensitive awareness and response to the way in which customers perceive their needs, both in consumer and industrial markets; and (2) an alertness to perceive how technological change will inevitably change the habits and ways of doing business of existing customers, opening new entrepreneurial opportunities in the areas still unperceived by the users themselves. This is a far different approach tobusiness and industry of health care (because of what has been termed "marketing myopia") characterized by product rather than customer orientation, and heavily locked into a company's or industry's existing technology (Heyel, C., 1972).

Redefinition of the basic function of the business in terms of customer need is the prime tenant of the "market concept" now increasingly discussed in professional marketing meetings and literature. It continually poses the question, "What is the customer really buying?" It is the kind of thinking that must be done by any farsighted management before it even begins to think about the direction its research diversification and acquisition program are to take.

Much of the new technology, particularly that part dealing with information processing, profoundly changes the manner in which health care is conducted. Companies must keep track of a number of fundamental areas of scientific work and must react rapidly to apply this work when the time is right. They must consciously plan to be the ones who obsolesces not only their own products, but their very industry.

REDESIGN OF PRODUCTS AND PROCESSES

The products and processes of health care must continually be reviewed, and often redesigned, to be sure the business will be able to meet new demands upon its systems. Health care organizations use new products requiring review. Design review must often be done before the new demands are even palpable. One of John Diebold's earliest and continuing major contribution to the developing concept of automation was his insistence that in order to make full use of technological innovation, it is usually necessary to redesign the product or process, or both (Heyel, C., 1972).

High tech digital products thread computer interface within a high-tech market industry citing smart clothing. One phototype of Georgia Tech Smart Fatigue is a special T-shirt designed by the U.S. Navy called "Sensate Liner." The Sensate Liner uses optical fibers to detect bullet wounds and special fibers to monitor vital signs during combat. The soldier attaches sensors to his body, pulls on the light weight shirt, then attaches the sensors to the shirt. The T-shirt functions like a computer, with plastic optical and conducting fibers woven throughout the fabric. A light signal is sent to a receiver if the receiver does not reach the receiver—the liner has been penetrated. Civilian applications for smart garments begin with police, fire and emergency crews. When incorporated into the design of infant pajamas, the Sensate technology can monitor the baby's respiration, alerting the parents of onset of Sudden Death Infant Syndrome (Page, D., 2000).

RETHINKING

Marketing Information Systems must be useful today and adaptable to the effective assimilation of future improvements, quantum mirage (Piller, C., 2000).

For some time now, new information systems have made substantial impact on health care as they have on accounting, production control, and the broad spectrum of administrative functions. Indeed, with the advent of remote access computers with large scale memories, hospitals have spent sizeable investments in developing technically impressive market data bases and information systems.

The implications of many of the technological developments alluded to raise issues of public policy for continued growth, if not sheer competitive survival. Individual enterprises must develop medical procedures for formalized technological forecasting of their own.

The imperatives of burgeoning technology in health care sends a signal to researchers to help develop over-the-horizon innovation. At first glance, medical research may be considered too far removed to have any discernible impact upon health care. A new approach, a new discipline; a new management function—already formalized in a few companies under the term technological forecasting—provides the necessary linkage between administrative, marketing, and financial decision makers. Accelerating technological developments of every sort, even those on the most far out fringes of science, can have a conceivable impact on the nature and function of the health care (Strauss, J. & Horlis, S., 1995).

HOSPITALS MUST COMPETE FOR BUSINESS

The growth and development of health care technology assessment (HCTA) reflect the need for informed technology decision making. HCTA is the evaluation of health care technology for its technical performance, safety, effectiveness, cost-effectiveness, and appropriate use. For many technologies, HCTA must address social, ethical, and legal implications as well (Goodman, C., 1997).

Although HCTA was originated largely by the government, HCTA is increasingly a private sector enterprise. HCTA can be used to identify instances of under use diagnostic technology as well as inappropriate diffusion of technology and must not reduce cost without regard to health outcome. About 90% of the health care dollar is spent on medical services, 8% is overhead.

The Health Care Financing Administration (HCFA), which will spend more than $200 billion in 1997 for some 39 million Medicare beneficiaries, has been slow to develop an HCTA capacity sufficient to meet the needs of the world's largest third party payer.

Coverage decisions for most procedures and other technologies are made by regional Medicare carriers reflecting regional practices and contributing to national variation in coverage policies.

HCTA methods are improving in several key areas, including primary data collection, synthesis methods, cost analyses and trials for data base settings, to examine the overall view of groups of patients in general practice.

Meta-analysis refers to a group of statistical techniques for combination of studies to conclude quantitative estimate of a particular intervention on a defined outcome. Thus combination may produce a stronger conclusion that can be provided by any individual study. Decision analysis uses data created by quantitative estimates to intervention strategies of probability for certain events, outcomes for patient population and associated costs of care (Goodman, C., 1997).

The current health care crisis in America reveals a significant need for improved performance and delivery of medical services. Through effective integration of design and technology, the fundamental objective of this research project is to reconceptualize, redesign, and design the Surgical Room of the Future ("SRF"). Implementation of research in high-tech innovation has far-reaching benefits in the context of administrative efficiency, procedural safety, and physical design. A tangible structure of the SRF prototype, has great potential for implementation in everyday life due to its predicted efficiency, versatility and its effectiveness in coordinating technical and medical interactions. To date, no other regional activities have proposed a medical facility of this type with special emphasis placed on collaboration between researchers, patients, health care providers, physicians, producers and manufacturers of medical equipment, and Virtual and Dynamic Environments ("VDE") (Durlach, N., 1994).

The essence of medical research is to developstate-of-the-art projects smart rooms. Outcomes:

1. The improvement of surgical efficiency by minimizing the complex physical and technological barriers between health care practitioners and equally complex surgical components;

2. The reduction of the hostile interface between patients, heath care providers, and surgical spaces; and

3. The enhancement of environments to augment automated surgical procedures.

The SRF represents the first attempt in the history of medical environment design to research and implement VE integration to health care facilities worldwide.

Long-term benefit from revolutionary design, surgical environment and procedural functionality can lead to long-term cost savings for state/federal governments, health care facilities, insurance companies, and the public. A unique advantage is the inherent sensitivity to patient-based needs for refined technical effectiveness, enhanced procedural efficiency, increased physical and psychological comfort, and reduced cost of surgical service (Goodman, C., 1997).

RECOMMENDATION: THE NEXT STEP

The Direct Approach (Gee, E. & Fine, A., 1997) means health care providers enter into direct contracting for several reasons—not all of them positive. A "top ten" list of current provider rationales for becoming involved in direct contracting:

1. Health maintenance organizations (HMOs) are making too much money.

2. Providers need to get higher up on the "food chain."

3. Providers have become nothing more than vendors in the health care delivery system.

4. Physicians are fed up with HMO executives making more than they do.

5. Providers have lost control of the market and do not like being out of control.

6. Managed care organizations (MCOs) do not really manage care, they manage cash.

7. Patients should have more choice in selecting physicians and hospitals.

8. Managed care system is inherently flawed because it encourages under utilization of service.

9. Manage care companies do not share the savings with the employers or providers.

10. Employers want to eliminate the intermediary function.

The three most important reasons that providers contract directly with health care providers are:

1. Direct contracting meets the need to regain and maintain contact with commercial customers (employers). In essence, it offers providers a vehicle for pursuing a meaningful partnership with purchasers of their services.

2. Direct contracting enables providers to prepare to deal directly with government purchasers for Medicare and Medicaid contracts.

3. Direct contracting aligns the incentives of hospitals and physicians with the reimbursement trends of the market place.

Hospitals need to spend resources and time to compete to survive. Simple. Partnerships with researchers offer promising financial rewards with alternative medical practice. The Surgical-angio Suite or the Surgical Room of the Future will provide a competitive edge. Long hospital stays are almost a medical practice of the past. Smart surgical procedures will ensure a "short day or so" hospital visit, intense patient care for a short period of time (Gee, E., & Fine, A., 1997).

U.S. research universities have received the largest federal grants, grossing $483 million from royalties on their inventions in fiscal 1997, up 44% from 1996. Of 132 U.S. universities, top earners (using adjusted gross income) were the University of California system, at $61.3 million; Columbia University, $46.1 million; Stanford University, $34 million; Florida State University, $29.9 million; and Massachusetts Institute of Technology, $19.9 million (Marklein, M., 1997).

The results come from the nonprofit Association of University Technology Managers (AUTM) whose members manage intellectual property resulting from discoveries in research institutions world-wide.

The survey which looked at 175 universities, teaching hospitals, research institutions in the USA and Canada, discovered that 4,267 new U.S. patents were filed by those organizations in fiscal 1997, up 31% from 1996, and 2,645 U.S.

patents were issued, up 26% from 1996. Among those approvals, Columbia University and a consortium of 13 companies last year patented a way to compress information to increase transmission capacity for use in high definition T.V. and other technology. This year Columbia University received the patent for the drug for glaucoma called Xalatan.

This is the seventh year AUTM has conducted the survey, designed to gauge the economic impact of research institutions. In fiscal year 1997, $28.7 billion of U.S. economic activity supporting 245,930 jobs, could be attributed to academic licensing, the report says. In 1996, $24.8 billion supported 212,000 jobs.

U.S. universities in 1997 executed 2,707 licenses and options, which led to the creation of 258 start-up companies, most in the same state as the university. Since 1980, 2,214 entrepreneurial ventures have been created to commercialize university technologies.

Most licensing has been in life sciences. Examples: hepatitis B vaccine by the University of California and Washington University; Retina A skin ointment, University of Pennsylvania; and chemotherapy for a type of leukemia, Brigham Young University. All have a direct impact on health care delivery (Marklein, M., 1997).

Beyond health care, these new tools will revolutionize economics through upwardly spiraling efficiencies in communications and transportation, material goods production and energy consumption. While there are obstacles, a path is becoming more clear that will lead us to a better health, more vibrant economies and more harmonious relationship with our planet's environment infrastructure. No doubt the time is now—find the perfect fit.

REFERENCES

Abele, J. Technology development from the perspective of industry. The Journal of Invasive Cardiology, V.5, No.2, (March 1993). Boston Scientific Corporation: Watertown, MA.

Ackerman, Ph.D. The visible human project. Bethesda, MD: Lister Hill National Center for Biomedical Communications, National Library of Medicine (1994).

Aday, L., Begley, C., Lairson, F., and Slater, C. Evaluating the medical care system: Efficacy, effectiveness, and equity. Ann Arbor, MI: Health Administration Press. (1993).

Advisory Board Company. The rising tide. Washington, D.C., (1996).

Ayers, J. & Benson, L. A road map for managed care success. Administrative Radiology Journal (August, 1995), pp.31-43.

Banter, H. Diffusion of minimally invasive therapy in Europe. Centre for Medical Technology, Netherlands organization for applied scientific research (1992).

Benso, L. & Ayers, J. A road map for managed care. Managed Care Edge (1995).

Bieze, A. The parties over—What's next for radiology? Diagnostic Imaging, December, 1995, pp.37-42.

Blonshine, S. "Eye on integration." Advance For Administrators in Radiology & Radiation Oncology (October, 1998), pp.15, 24.

Boland, P., Ph.D. Making Managed Healthcare Work. "A Practical Guide to Strategies and Solutions. Aspen Publishers, Inc. (1993), pp. 6-25.

Brook, R., & Lohr, K. Efficacy, effectiveness, various and quality: Boundary-crossing research. Medical Care, 23 (1985), pp.710-722.

Burrow, M. A telemedicine test bed for developing and evaluating tele-robotic tools for rural health care. Medicine Meets Virtual Reality II Interactive Technology (January, 1994), UCSD, San Diego, pp.15-20.

Calkins, D., Fernandopulle, R., & Marino, B. (1995). Health care policy. Cambridge, MA: Blackwell Science Incorporated (1995).

Champy, J. Reengineering management: The mandate for new leadership. Harper Business (1995).

Chan, G. Robodoc maker enters middle eastern market. The Sacramento Bee (January 9, 1999), A1 & C2.

Chandler, D. Supercold jar incubates a superatom." The Sacramento Bee (Friday, July 14, 1995) p1 + 19.

Charles, S., M.D. Dexterity enhancement in microsurgery using telemicro-robotics. Medicine Meets Virtual Reality II Interactive Technology (January, 1994), UCSD, San Diego, pp.19-20.

Connect, The Weekly Newsletter of UCSD Connect. Forum interfaces medicine and VR to create the future of medical treatment (Tuesday, January 20, 1998, Issues 8-3).

Davis, J. The future of major ambulatory surgery. Surg Clin North Am, 67 (1997), pp.893-901.

Deutsch, D., and Ekert, A. Quantum Communication Moves Into The Unknown. Extract from Physic world. (June, 1993).

Ditlea, S. "The PC you wear." Popular Mechanics (December, 1998), pp.54-57.

Doyle, D., Ph.D., Noe, A., Ph.D., Carlloom, I., Ph.D., Ang, C., M.S., & Martin, D., M.S. The virtual embryo: VR applications in human development anatomy. Medicine Meets Virtual Reality II Interactive Technology (January, 1994), UCSD, San Diego, pp.38-41.

Dumay, A. C. M. Cybersurgery. Medicine Meets Virtual Reality II Interactive Technology (January, 1994), UCSD, San Diego, pp.42-44.

Durlach, N. <u>Psychophysical considerations in the design of human-machine interfaces for teleoperator and virtual-environment systems</u>. Virtual Environment and Teleoperator Research Consortium (VETREC): Massachusetts Institute of Technology: Cambridge, MA (1994).

EDRI Outpatient Surgery: It's Perils and Prospects. <u>Health Technology</u>, 1:91-8 (1989).

Elliot, J. Trinity hospital uses system integration to provide better health care with telemedicine. <u>Applied Radiology</u>, (February, 1998), pp.33-37.

Epstein, J. & Axtell, J. Sugarscape: Tierra. <u>Science News</u> (November 23, 1996).

Fang-Fany, Y., Ph.D. <u>Advance For Administrators In Radiology & Radiation Oncology</u> (October, 1998), pp. 38, 40-44.

Ford, K. & Hayes, P. On computational wings, rethinking the goals of artificial intelligence. <u>California Computer News</u> (Sept., 2000).

Gallon, C. C., M.D., Ph.D. Neuromagnetic functional brain mapping. <u>Medicine Meets Virtual Reality II Interactive Technology</u> (January, 1994), UCSD, San Diego, pp.59-62.

Gcc, E. & Fine, A. The direct approach. <u>Health Systems Review</u> (1997), 70, 72, 74.

Gibbons, M. Regulating research: Experimentation on humans still raises ethical concerns. <u>Advance For Radiology Science Professionals</u>, Vol XI, No. 22 (October 26, 1998), pp.31-33.

Gingrich, N. To renew America. <u>Harper Collins Publishers</u>, (1995).

Ginsberg, M. Computers, games and the real world. <u>Scientific American</u> (Sept., 1995).

Glausiusz, J. Future tech—spare parts. <u>Discover</u>, Vol. 20, No. 8 (August, 1999), pp.13-16.

Golden, F. & Lemonick, M. The race is over. <u>Time</u> (July 3, 2000), pp.19-23.

Goodman, C. S. Closer inspection: The recent evolution of technology assessment. Health Systems Review (March/April, 1997), pp.38-56.

Gott, III, R. "Will we travel in time?" Time (April 10, 2000), p.80.

Greenleaf, W. J., Ph.D. Data glove and data suit—virtual reality technology applied to the measurement of human movement. Medicine Meets Virtual Reality II Interactive Technology (January, 1994), UCSD, San Diego, pp.63-69.

Griffith, D. Sutter Cancer Center installs a gamma knife. The Sacramento Bee, (August 2, 1998).

Hamilton, D. It may sound like science fiction but the next leap in computing will be a quantum one. Northern California, Vol. 6 (September, 2000), p.24, 28, 30, & 34.

Hatfield, S. Spiral CT and virtual reality help plan less-invasive procedures. Advance For Radiologic Science Professionals (September 8, 1997), pp.6-7.

Hatfield, S. The many sides of CT. Advance For Radiologic Science Professionals (September 14, 1998), pp.14-17.

Hatfield, S. Intraoperative CT, Advance For Administrators In Radiology And Radiation Oncology (October, 1998), pp.51-52.

Hatfield, S. Multidisciplinary approaches will help keep radiology at the forefront of interventional medicine. Advance For Radiologic Science Professionals, Vol. XI, No. 22 (October 26, 1998), pp.9-10.

Hatfield, S. New developments in radiology. Advance For Radiologic Science Professionals (November 23, 1998), pp.10-12.

Hatfield, S. Ashes to ashes. Advance For Radiologic Science Professionals, Vol. 12 (January 25, 1999), pp.8-9, 12-13.

Hatfield, S. Imaging and interventions. Advance For Radiologic Science Professionals, Vol. 12 (January 25, 1999), pp.12-13.

Havanaugh-Brown, J. Creating the future of technology. <u>California Computer News</u>, Vol. XVI (January, 1999), pp.24-35.

Hayden, M. <u>Human genome project</u>—Cal Tech. University of Columbia (1998).

Hayes, E. Managed-care inpatients receive fewer imaging tests. <u>Diagnostic Imaging</u> (December, 1996), pp.11-13.

<u>Health Systems Review</u>. National Association of Psychiatric Health Systems (1996), Annual Survey Report.

Heyel, C. <u>John Diebold on management</u>. Princeton, New Jersey: Van Nostrand Company (1972).

Hon, D., President, Ixion, Inc. Ixion's laparoscopic surgical skills simulator. <u>Medicine Meets Virtual Reality II Interactive Technology</u> (January, 1994), UCSD, San Diego, pp.81-89.

Hunter, I. Teleoperated microsurgical robot and associated virtual environment. <u>Medicine Meets Virtual Reality II Interactive Technology</u> (January, 1994), UCSD, San Diego, pp.85-89.

Johnson, S., Ph.D. & Hadley, S. Setting sights on computer vision. <u>Computer Mechanics</u> (December, 1998), pp.30-48.

Kaker, M. What will replace silicon? <u>Time</u> (June 19, 2000), pp.98-99.

Kaplan, K. L. Project description: Surgical room of the future. <u>Interactive Technology & Health Care</u> (January 1994), pp.95-98.

Kasler, D. Technology of the year. <u>Applied Radiology</u> (February, 1998), p.37.

Kasler, D.Chips and DNA dip. <u>The Sacramento Bee</u> (March 29, 1999), p.15.

Kaufman, L, Ph.D. Real reality: Being there with open access MRI. <u>Medicine Meets Virtual Reality II Interactive Technology</u> (January, 1994), UCSD, San Diego, pp.99-102.

Kelly, P. J., M.D. Quantitative virtual reality surgical simulation, minimally invasive stereotactic neurosurgery and frameless stereotactics technologies.

Medicine Meets Virtual Reality II Interactive Technology (January, 1994), UCSD, San Diego, pp.103-108.

Komando, K. "Technology: Inside the new Pentium III." Popular Mechanics (May, 1999), pp. 38-40.

Konigsmark, A. R. "Stanford expects medical miracles with dream teams. San Jose Mercury News (October 5, 2000), www.Mercury center.com.

Kormos, D. W., Ph.D. Wandering through the body: Modern computer-assisted surgery. Medicine Meets Virtual Reality II Interactive Technology (January, 1994), UCSD, San Diego, pp.109-112.

Krushenisky, C. "Smart Computing." Technology News (November, 1997) pp. 4-5.

Kuhnapfel, U. G. Real time graphical computer simulation for endoscopic surgery. Medicine Meets Virtual Reality II Interactive Technology (January, 1994), UCSD, San Diego, pp.111-116.

Kyes, K. Excerpts from a virtual symposium. The Journal Of Imaging Technology, Vol. 11, No. 5 (September/October 1998), pp.51-68.

Lateiner, J. S. The Vox-L stereoscopic workstation: Stereoscopic interactive volume visualization for medical data. Medicine Meets Virtual Reality II Interactive Technology (January, 1994), UCSD, San Diego, pp.117-120.

Lau, E. New bionic chip may really bring gene therapy to life. The Sacramento Bee (February 25, 2000), pp. 1, 26.

Lenat, D. Artificial intelligence. Scientific American (Sept. 1995).

Le Postollec, M. "Bridging the culture gap." Advance For Radiologic Science Professionals (September 14, 1998), p.39.

Lorensen, W., M.S. Enhancing reality in the operating room. Medicine Meets Virtual Reality II Interactive Technology (January, 1994), UCSD, San Diego, pp.124-127.

Luden, The Netherlands, Popular Science (August 1998), p.12.

Marklein, M. "Research universities boost economy." U.S.A. Today (February 1998).

Martinez, R., Ph.D. Remote consultation and diagnosis via the global medical informatic consortium networks. Medicine Meets Virtual Reality II Interactive Technology (January, 1994), UCSD, San Diego, pp.140-143.

Mases, P. Intelligent software. Scientific American (Sept. 1995).

Matthews, R., M.S.C. The information highway: European efforts toward a multi-media health care infrastructure. Medicine Meets Virtual Reality II Interactive Technology (January, 1994), UCSD, San Diego, pp.144-149.

McGovern, K. T. The virtual clinic TM—a virtual reality surgical simulator. Medicine Meets Virtual Reality II Interactive Technology (January, 1994), UCSD, San Diego, pp.150-157.

Merrill, J. R., M.D. Surgeon on the cutting edge—virtual reality applications in medical education. Virtual Reality World (November/December, 1993).

National Library of Medicine (U.S.) Board of Regents. Electronic imaging. Report of the Board of Regents (U.S. Department of Health and Human Services, Public Health Service, National Institute of Health: (1990) N.H. Publication 90-2197.

National Library of Medicine's Website: www.rlm.rib.gov/research/invisible/.

Ogle, P. "Imaging." Diagnostic Imaging (1996), p.5, 11, 13.

O'Shanghnessy, K. "The visible human project." Advance for Radiologic Science Professionals (January 31, 2000), pp.30-31.

Page, D. Wearware: One device fits all. California Computer News, Vol. XVII (October, 2000), p. 18 & 19. www.CCNMAG.com.

Peltz, J. Virtual humans for profit, research. San Francisco Examiner (November 29, 1998), B1.

Pentland, A. Wearable intelligence. Scientific American (1995).

Piller, C. Move over, microprocessor: Circuitry goes atomic. The Sacramento Bee, (Thursday, February 3, 2000), p.9.

Poston, T. & Serra, L. The medical reality sculptor. Medicine Meets Virtual Reality II Interactive Technology (January, 1994), UCSD, San Diego, pp.174-176.

Poulos, C. Defining tomorrow's information. California Computer News, Vol. XV (May, 1998), p.48.

Popular Science. What's New—Ultracision (August, 1998), p.12.

Porter, M. Competitive strategy: techniques for analyzing industry and competitors. New York: Free Press (1980).

Porter, M. How competitive forces shape strategy. Harvard Business Review, 57, No. 2 (March-April, 1979).

Quantum Teleportation. IBM Research. IBM Corporation (1996).

Reddick, E., & Olsen, D. Outpatient laparoscopic laser cholecystectomy. American Journal of Surgery, 160 (199), pp.485-487.

Romans, L. E., R.T., (R)(CT). PACS. Computed Tomograph (1997).

Rosen, J. M. The role of telemedicine and telepresence in reducing health care costs. Medicine Meets Virtual Reality II Interactive Technology (January, 1994), UCSD, San Diego, pp.187-199.

Rubin, R. Industry's rapid growth, change defy regulation. USA Today (November 2, 1998).

Sandsmark, F. Does your doctor make house calls? California Computer News, Vol. XVII (January, 2000), pp.48-49.

Sandsmark, F. Computer trials at Internet Speeds. California Computer News, Vo. XVII (September, 2000), www.comm66.com.

Sandsmark, F. The Web is accelerating and improving of new medical treatments. California Computer News (Sept. 2000), pp. 20 & 21.

Schaffer, D. L., M.D. What is imaging's role in managed-care world? <u>Diagnostic Imaging</u> (December 1995), pp.31-38.

Schilling, R., Ph.D. Framework facilitiates assessment of Paces. <u>Diagnostic Imaging</u> (December, 1995), pp.55-64.

Schuller, R. <u>Success is never ending, failure is never final</u>. New York: Thomas Nelson Publishers, (1988), p.191.

Seebach-Persico, J. Managed implementation. <u>Medical Information & Management Systems</u> (May/June, 1997), pp.5-7.

Smith, Brad. Vital Signs Stealth Station Improves Doctor's Surgical Vision. <u>The Denver Business Journal</u>: Denver, Colorado (April 7, 1997).

Smith, K, D.Sc., Frank, K. J., M.S., & Bucholz, R., M.D. The neurostation TM applications to minimally invasive neurosurgery. <u>Medicine Meets Virtual Reality II Interactive Technology</u> (January, 1994), UCSD, San Diego, pp.209-211.

Smith, K., D.Sc., Frank, K., M.S. & Bucholz, R., M.D. <u>The neuro station—applications to minimally invasive neurosurgery</u>. Marine, Illinois: Stealth, Inc. (1994).

Smith, K. E-Mail Krs.minuet.siw, edu. Stealth Technologies, Inc. (1999).

Smith, R. "Cost-effectiveness for value." <u>Imaging Economics</u> (Sept/Oct. 1998), Vol. 11, No. 5, pp. 22, 24, 31, 38, 46.

<u>Spectrum</u>. "The PC goes ready to wear." (October, 2000), Vol. 37, No. 10, pp.34-39.

Stephenson, J., Ph.D. Human genome project on fast track. <u>Journal Of The American Medical Association</u>, Vol. 280, No. 15 (October 21, 1998), p.1298.

Steven, P. "Dicom Standards." <u>Advance For Administrators in Radiology</u> (February, 1997), pp. 52-53.

Stover, D. Growing hearts from scratch. <u>Popular Science</u> (April 2000), pp.47-50.

Stredney, D. Virtual simulations through high performance computing. <u>Medicine Meets Virtual Reality II Interactive Technology</u> (January, 1994), UCSD, San Diego, pp.212-215.

Sukthankar, M. S. & Reddy, N., Ph.D. Towards virtual reality of tissue squeezing: A feasibility study. <u>Medicine Meets Virtual Reality II Interactive Technology</u> (January, 1994), UCSD, San Diego, pp.182-184.

Strauss, J. & Horli, S., M.D. Imaging in the new millennium. <u>Medical Imaging 2095</u>, Fuji Medical Systems, Hospital of the University of Pennsylvania (August, 1998), pp.41-43.

Surgical Navigator Technologies. <u>Stealth Station Treatment Guidance Platform: A New Area in Surgical Navigation and Information</u> (1997).

<u>Surgery Clinic North America</u>. The Future of Major Ambulatory Surgery, 67 (1987), pp.893-901.

Tamas, M. J. Radiology industry profile: Industry-wide effort forms to accelerate plug-and-play interoperatbility in health care. <u>Advance For Administrators In Radiology</u> (February, 1997), p.52; p.58.

Taubes, G. Tech watch. <u>UCLA Magazine</u> (Spring 2000) uclastore.com, pp.24-25; p.45.

Taubes, G. Speed demon. <u>UCLA Magazine</u> (Spring 2000), pp. 23, 24, 25, 45.

Technology of the Year. (February, 1998). Applied Radiology, p.37.

Tokita, J. One World One Language. <u>California CCN Computer News</u>, Vol. XVI, 35 (April, 1999).

Van Nostrand Company, Inc. <u>Automation: The Advent of the Automatic Factory</u>. Princeton, Jew Jersey (1952).

Van Winkle, W. Will technology create artificial life? <u>California Computer News</u>, Vol. XV (May, 1998) www.cnnmag.com, p.57.

Vondeling, H., Kievits, V., & Schoul, B. Palliation of advanced colon cancer. <u>Lasers in Health Care</u>, Copenhagen Academic Publishing (1991), pp.140-147.

Waitley, D. The double win. <u>Fleming H. Revell Co</u> (1985).

Ward, J. CN MT, RT (N). Surgical options for brain tumors. <u>Advance For Radiologic Science Professionals</u> (June 8, 1998), pp.14-16.

Ward, J., CNMT, RT(N). Imaging at the speed of CT. <u>Advance For Radiologic Science Professionals</u> (September 14, 1998), pp.12-16.

Ward, J. CN MT, RT (N). Making waves in the operating room. <u>Advance For Radiologic Science Professions</u> (October 26, 1998), pp.14-15.

Ward, J., CN MT, R(N). Computer monitor: Info rad. <u>Advance For Radiologic Science Professionals</u> (November 23, 1998), p.8.

Ward, J., CN MT, R(N). CT or MRI in OR. <u>Advance For Radiologic Science Professionals</u> (November 23, 1998), pp. 34-35.

Ward, J., CN MT, RT (N). Radiology gives surgeons new tools. <u>Advance For Radiologic Science</u>, Vol. 11, No. 25 (December 7, 1998), pp.16-17.

Ward, J. CM NT, RT(N). Fluoroscopy & CT. <u>Advance For Radiologic Science Professionals</u>, Vol. 12 (June 14, 1999), pp.16-17; p.29.

Ward, J. Multiple modalities better than one. <u>Advance For Radiologic Science Professionals</u> (January 31, 2000), pp.13-16.

Ward, J. Watching the mind in action. <u>Advance For Radiologic Science Professionals</u> (January 21, 2000), pp.13-14.

Weber, T. E. "E-world—a doctor to patients on the net: Inventing the virtual housecall. <u>The Wall Street Journal</u> (Monday, January 17, 2000).

Wenzlick, P. "Panning for gold at HIMSS." <u>Health Systems Review</u> (March/April, 1997), pp. 12, 14-15, 22, 27-28.

Wiederhold, M.D., Ph.D. <u>Neural networks in medical diagnosis</u>. La Jolla, California: Division of Internal Medicine, Scripps Clinic and Research Foundation (1995).

Wilson, J. Beam me up. <u>Computer Mechanics</u> (December, 1998), pp.72-73.

Wilson, J. Technology watch: Big hopes for tiny machines. <u>Popular Mechanics</u> (August, 1999), p.21.

Yam, P. Intelligence considered. <u>Scientific American</u>, pp.10-11.

Yee, S. Get wired. <u>Advance For Administrators In Radiology and Radiation Oncolgy</u>, Volume 10, No. 2 (February, 2000), pp.6-11, 34-37.

Zey, M., Ph.D. <u>Seizing the future</u>. New York: Simon & Schuster (1994).

0-595-29644-0

www.ingramcontent.com/pod-product-compliance
Lightning Source LLC
Chambersburg PA
CBHW021004180526
45163CB00005B/1891